Guide to Basic Electrocardiography

Guide to Basic Electrocardiography

John Wagner Beasley, M.D., and
E. Wayne Grogan, Jr., M.D.

University of Wisconsin Medical School
Madison, Wisconsin

PLENUM MEDICAL BOOK COMPANY • NEW YORK AND LONDON

Library of Congress Cataloging-in-Publication Data

Beasley, John Wagner.
Guide to basic electrocardiography / John Wagner Beasley and E. Wayne Grogan, Jr.
p. cm.
Includes bibliographical references.
Includes index.
ISBN-13:978-0-306-43296-5 e-ISBN-13:978-1-4613-0517-0
DOI:10.1007/978-1-4613-0517-0

1. Electrocardiography. [1. Electrocardiography.] I. Grogan, E. Wayne. II. Title.
[DNLM: WG 140 B368g]
RC683.5.E5B375 1990
616.1'2'07547--dc20
DNLM/DLC
for Library of Congress 90-7327
CIP

233 Spring Street, New York, N.Y. 10013

Plenum Medical Book Company is an imprint of Plenum Publishing Corporation

Preface

The purpose of this text is to provide a reference work covering basic electrocardiographic (ECG) patterns and diagnoses in a succinct and useful format. The book covers common adult ECG abnormalities and is organized according to the type of abnormality, rather than by specific disease or ECG diagnosis. Detailed lists of possible causes for various ECG patterns have been included wherever appropriate, and particular attention has been paid to the diagnosis of common rhythm problems.

The contents are directed at the primary physician in residency training or in practice, and a reasonable background knowledge of terminology and basic pathophysiology is assumed. Thus, certain topics, such as a detailed discussion of electrophysiology, are omitted for the sake of brevity. For a discussion of this topic, complex or unusual rhythm patterns, and the advanced techniques of deciphering unusual rhythms and other uncommon abnormalities, the reader is referred to other, more detailed, texts. The techniques of performing an ECG are not covered here and the topic of children's ECGs is treated only briefly. A number of more detailed self-study and reference texts are available, which the authors have found useful in the preparation of this text and in their clinical work.[1–5]

The ECG tracings included here as examples have generally been selected as common examples of abnormalities, often as they occur in concert with other abnormalities, rather than as pure "classic" examples of a single abnormality. Therefore, in many instances the examples given include commonly associated abnormalities in addition to the one under discussion. They are thus representative of the reality of clinical practice, where abnormalities only occasionally occur in their pure, isolated, and classical forms.

Contents

1

Introduction

At rest, the cells of the myocardium, like other cells, have a positive charge on the outer surface and a negative charge inside the cell. When the myocardium is at rest, there is no deflection in any electrocardiographic (ECG) lead since all the cells, and thus the surfaces of the heart (both epicardial and endocardial), maintain a positive surface charge.

However, when depolarization takes place, some cells (those not yet affected by the wave of depolarization) maintain their positive surface charges, while others (those which have undergone depolarization) have lost theirs, thus giving rise to an electrical gradient. Since the myocardium depolarizes from the inside outward (that is, from the endocardium to the epicardium), the epicardial surface of the myocardium assumes a relative positive charge as it undergoes depolarization.

Thus, during the phase of depolarization (the P wave for the atria and the QRS complex for the ventricles), the inside of the heart remains relatively negative and those leads "looking" at a particular surface of the heart will, by convention, "see" a positive deflection during depolarization.

In the case of a transmural myocardial infarction (which creates an area of electrical inactivity or an "electrical hole" in the myocardium) the lead "looking" at that portion of the myocardium "sees" through the inactive myocardium to the negative interior of the heart. This gives rise to the typical negative deflection (the Q wave) seen in that lead overlying the area of infarction.

Repolarization of the myocardium takes place in a sequence opposite to that of depolarization, thus giving rise to a T wave which is usually positive in the same lead. However, while the electrical axis of the T wave is roughly the same as the QRS axis, there may be significant differences even in normal hearts, especially in children.

Acute injury to the myocardium gives rise to a steady state of positivity on the myocardial surface (the epicardium) during the period between depolarization and repolarization, and thus an elevated ST segment is seen in the leads looking at that portion of the surface of the heart where injury occurs.

2

A Way to Visualize the Electrocardiogram in Relation to the Heart

There is an easy way to visualize the electrocardiographic (ECG) pattern that will be seen by any particular lead. This is done by making a rough model of the heart on your own chest wall, from which the relationship of the underlying heart to the various ECG leads can be visualized.

Your left hand is held over your precordium, with the fist loosely clenched and the thumb upward. The plane defined by the backs of the proximal phalanges should be at an angle of about 30° from the vertical angling toward a point slightly above your left iliac crest. Now your right hand is placed loosely over the left, with the right palm and fingers overlying the proximal phalanges and knuckles of the left hand. You now have represented the left ventricle with your left hand, the interventricular septum with the proximal phalanges of your left hand, and the right ventricle with your overlying right hand. The left thumb represents the aorta and the right thumb the pulmonary artery. This is shown in Figure 1.

Now you can, for example, visualize the "view" of the heart which aVL will "see" by imagining that aVL is "looking" inward from the left shoulder. In the same manner you can visualize limb lead I "looking" inward from about the 5th interspace at the left midaxillary line, limb lead II from near the left costal margin in the same line, aVF from the left leg, limb lead III from near the right costal margin, and aVR from the right shoulder.

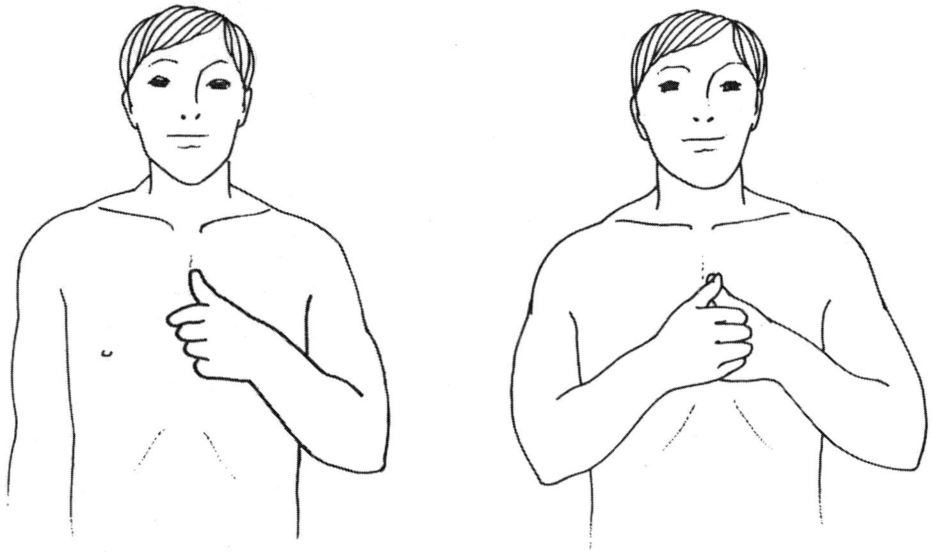

Figure 1. A method of visualizing the heart within the thoracic cavity (see text for details).

Figures 2 and 3 show the relationship of the heart in the body of the view "seen" by the limb leads and to the determination of the electrical axis in the frontal plane. The relationship of the precordial leads to the simulated heart is self-evident.

For example, consider the events that aVL will "see" when the normal heart depolarizes. The first ventricular event is depolarization of the septum (represented by the proximal phalanges of the left hand), which, since it proceeds from left to right, will most often be seen as a small negative deflection; the small septal Q often seen in aVL. Next, the large mass of left ventricular muscle will depolarize from the inside outward, giving rise to a positive deflection (the R wave). If the conduction to the free wall of the right ventricle occurs after the large and overwhelming events of the left ventricle are over, a small S wave arising from aVL's view of the depolarization of the right ventricular free wall will also be seen.

To continue to explore this model, consider what will happen if there is a marked delay in right ventricular depolarization as occurs with right bundle branch block (RBBB). aVL will "see," late in the depolarization cycle, the electrical forces originating from the back of the right ventricular wall, which will result in an abnormally large, delayed terminal S wave in aVL (as well as in lead I and the lateral precordial leads).

Similarly, imagine what will be "seen" by V6 if the septum is abnormally large (as in idiopathic hypertrophic subaortic stenosis) and thus generates abnormally large septal forces. These may appear as abnormally large Q waves in V6 and must be differentiated from the Q waves of lateral-wall myocardial infarction.

As a final example, imagine the events "seen" by V1 when RBBB is present. The first deflection will be from the depolarization of the septum and will, since it travels from left to right, be positive. This gives rise to the common and normal initial R wave in V1. The next event will be an S wave resulting from this lead "looking" at depolarization of the mass of the left ventricle. Finally, a terminal R wave will result from the delayed and unopposed depolarization of the right ventricular wall.

This model has the advantage of allowing visu-

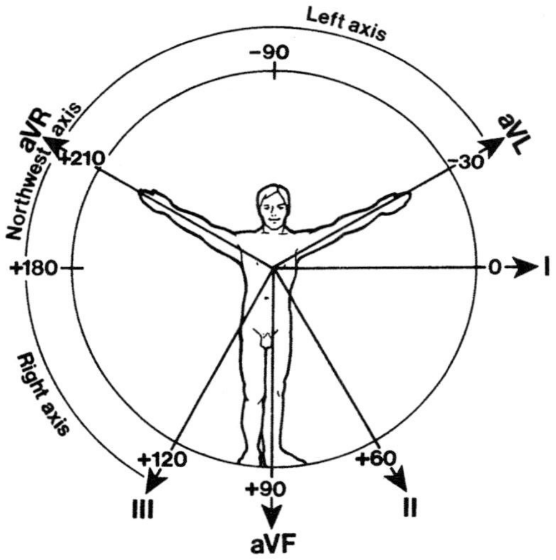

Figure 2. A method of visualizing the standard frontal plane leads with respect to the human body.

alization of the different ECG patterns that result from changes in cardiac position. For example, these may occur in the patient with severe chronic obstructive pulmonary disease, in whom the heart has a more vertical axis as it hangs down in the hyperinflated chest; or, by contrast, in the very obese patient where the heart will be rotated to a more horizontal position owing to the elevated diaphragm.

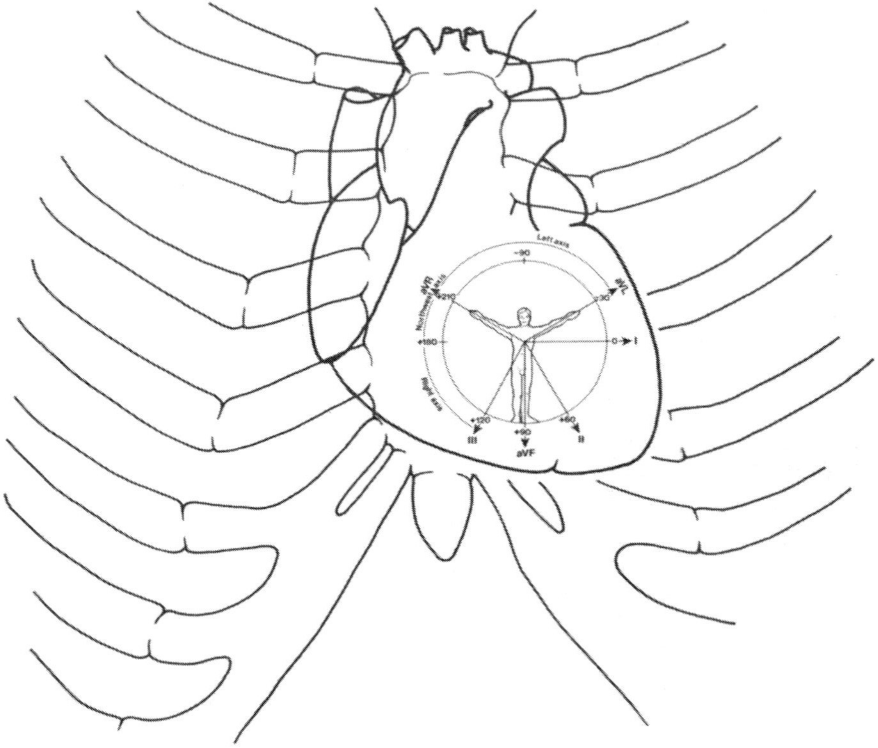

Figure 3. A method of visualizing the standard frontal plane leads with respect to the heart within the thorax.

3

The Formal Reading of the Electrocardiogram

INTRODUCTION

To make a formal reading of the electrocardiogram (ECG), data regarding the patient are required. The minimal data set should include:

1. Age of the patient
2. Height and weight
3. Known medical problems
4. Medications
5. Reason for performing the ECG

Any previous ECGs should be available. As is the case with most diagnostic studies in medicine, the more information available about the clinical status of the patient and the reason for performing the study, the more useful the ECG interpretation will be.

The formal reading of the ECG may be divided into two components: description and interpretation.

THE DESCRIPTION OF THE ELECTROCARDIOGRAM

The description of an ECG should be given in enough detail that a person reading it will have at least a rough mental image of the ECG even if the actual tracing is not available. The description should not contain interpretations of the tracing, but rather should describe what is there. A complete, stepwise description of the tracing will help to avoid errors in interpretation. The description should give the following details:

1. The atrial rate
2. The ventricular rate
3. The rhythm
4. The intervals (P–R, QRS, Q–T)
5. The axis (in degrees, not just "normal" or "abnormal"); at times the axis is indeterminate and no specific axis can be given
6. A description of the P waves
7. A description of the QRS complexes to include presence or absence of Q waves, whether such Q waves are normal or abnormal, the R-wave progression, the voltages if abnormal, and any conduction abnormalities, such as slurring, delta waves, or bundle branch block

8. A description of the ST segments (isoelectric or otherwise)
9. A description of the T waves, including normal variants
10. A description of U waves if present
11. A description of this ECG relative to any previous tracings

THE ANATOMY OF THE NORMAL TRACING (Fig. 4)

The anatomy of the normal P-QRS-T is shown in Figure 4.

The easiest way to calculate the heart rate is to divide the number of large lines between the peaks of two typical R waves into 300. This is because the interval between any two of the heavy lines on the ECG is 0.20 sec and thus the paper will traverse five heavy lines in 1 sec and 300 heavy lines in 1 min. For greatest accuracy, one can determine a 6-sec period, count the number of R waves in that period, and multiply by 10. For most purposes, the former method is faster and of sufficient precision.

Usually it is sufficient to give the Q–T interval without correction for rate unless the rate is much different from 60. However, since the Q–T interval varies with rate, if the rate is much different from 60 (especially if it is clinically indicated), it is necessary to calculate the corrected Q–T interval or Q–Tc (see Chapter 6 for the method of calculation of the corrected Q–T interval).

The upper limits of normal for the intervals are as follows:

P–R: 0.20 sec for the P–R interval (0.21 if rate is less than 70 in a large adult); these limits are lower in children and when higher heart rates are present

QRS: 0.08 sec in small children to 0.10 sec in adults

Intrinsicoid deflection: 0.05 sec in the lateral precordial leads

Q–Tc: 0.42 sec (men) or 0.43 sec (women) in adults

The electrical axis in the frontal plane can be simply determined with sufficient precision by the following method. First, find the lead in the frontal plane (I, II, III, aVR, aVL, or aVF) that is most nearly isoelectric (or a point between two leads that would, by interpolation, appear to be). In deciding this, estimate the area of the QRS complex under and above the baseline, not just the height and depth of the QRS complex. The axis lies at roughly 90° to this lead, and it is simple to determine whether it is to the right or left of this isoelectric lead by simply noting on which side the complexes are predominantly positive. There are times when there is no prominent axis in the frontal plane, and thus the axis must be read as "indeterminate."

The terms "right axis" and "left axis" are somewhat inconsistent with the frontal plane in which they are described. It would be more accurate to use the terms "superior axis" and "inferior axis," but that is not the convention and the usual terms of "right" and "left" axis are used here.

THE INTERPRETATION OF THE ELECTROCARDIOGRAM

The interpretation of the ECG should state directly whether it is normal, abnormal, or, rarely, borderline. It is always possible to add qualifiers to the statement "normal" if the changes are minor. If abnormal or borderline, the interpretation should state the basis for this. The reader must bear in mind that although diagnostic accuracy is needed, as much harm can be done to a patient through an overly aggressive interpretation as through an overly conservative one. An example would be calling a tracing with a normal bradycardia, minor T-wave changes, or an incomplete right bundle branch block "abnormal." It will serve the patient just as well to interpret the tracing as "normal with incidental . . . noted." In some instances, especially with ST- and T-wave changes that are nondiagnostic, it will be necessary to suggest that a follow-up tracing be done to determine whether the changes are chronic and stable or represent an acute process.

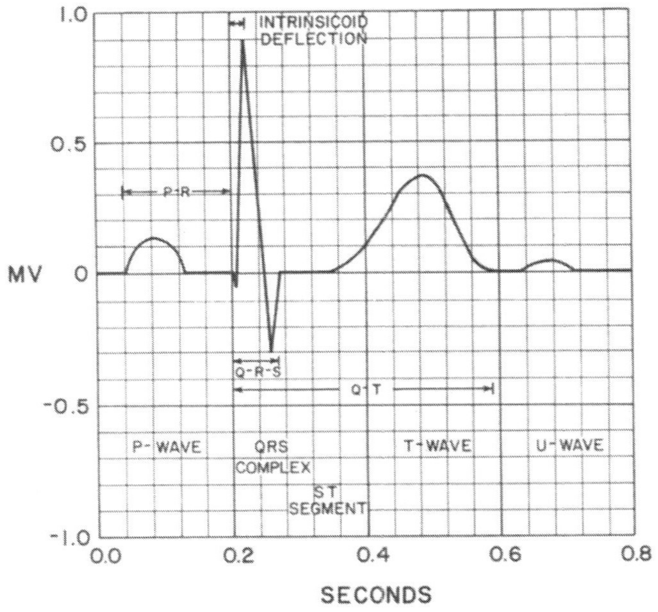

Figure 4. The normal cardiac cycle as seen on the electrocardiogram.

4

Indications for Performing an Electrocardiogram

INTRODUCTION

Probably few diagnostic tests have been as overutilized as the electrocardiogram (ECG). It is often assumed that the ECG, perhaps as the modern "high-tech" equivalent of chicken entrails, enables the high priests of medicine to foretell the future of the patient. This nearly magical quality ascribed to the ECG should not be ignored, as it may create disease where none is present, reassure falsely, or even be a healing force. It has been demonstrated that patients in emergency rooms with noncardiac chest pain recover more rapidly if an ECG is done.[6] However, it must be remembered that the resting ECG has little value in predicting the risk of subsequent development of cardiac disease in the individual patient, particularly the development of events related to coronary artery disease.

SCREENING

The routine resting ECG is of minimal use as a screening test, having high false positive and false negative rates for coronary artery disease as well as most other diseases. Up to 2% of otherwise healthy persons between 18 and 25 years of age have ECG abnormalities exclusive of technical errors.[7] There is no evidence that a "baseline" ECG has sufficient clinical usefulness to warrant doing one routinely in asymptomatic patients. Nonetheless, as mentioned earlier, patients may feel reassured when told that their ECG is normal, and in some circumstances it may be necessary to do one simply to meet patient expectations. Even the exercise ECG has significant limitations as a screening tool in asymptomatic patients owing to false positives and false negatives.

HYPERTENSION

It is rare that ECG findings will alter the course of treatment for hypertension since the treatment will depend primarily on measured blood pressures and other clinical factors. There is little justification for doing ECGs routinely in hypertensive patients, particularly in patients with earlier and milder forms of the disease where cardiac abnormalities related to the blood pressure are uncommon. However, the finding of ECG evidence of left ventricular hypertrophy may provide corroborating evidence that a patient has had significant, long-standing elevation of the arterial pressure.

CORONARY ARTERY DISEASE, CHEST PAIN, AND ISCHEMIA

The ECG is not very useful as a screening tool for coronary artery disease unless acute symptoms are present, whereas the presence of diagnostic ECG abnormalities during episodes of chest pain is very helpful in diagnosing myocardial ischemia. However, the ECG may be normal even in the presence of ischemic pain, and *a normal ECG does not exclude myocardial ischemia*. To further complicate the picture, changes in the ECG suggestive of ischemia can occur with anxiety, hyperventilation, or as a normal variant. Overall, however, the ECG is essential in the diagnosis of acute myocardial infarction (MI), and rapid recording and interpretation of the ECG are helpful in diagnosing MI and selecting patients for thrombolytic or other appropriate therapies for acute MI.

As a measure of past ischemic damage to the heart, the ECG has some limitations. Up to 30% of persons who have had documented MIs may lose the original Q waves within the first year. In addition, there are many patients who experience non-Q-wave infarctions, characterized by changes in ST segments and T waves but not the development of Q waves. Thus, although the presence of characteristic Q waves on the ECG can be very helpful in diagnosing old MI, the absence of such findings does not exclude old infarction.

PERICARDITIS AND MYOCARDITIS

The ECG is useful in the diagnosis of pericarditis. Pericarditis is initially manifested on the ECG as widespread ST segment elevation. However, the ECG changes seen in patients with myocarditis and the cardiomyopathies are of limited diagnostic use. This is because these changes are inconsistent and of a wide variety. They include left ventricular hypertrophy, pseudoinfarction patterns, bundle branch blocks, arrhythmias, and nonspecific ST- and T-wave changes.

PALPITATIONS, SYNCOPE, AND ARRHYTHMIAS

The standard ECG is of minimal usefulness unless the arrhythmia is present at the time that it is being taken. In fact, the ECG may well be falsely reassuring since serious rhythm disturbances may occur so episodically that they are hard to capture on a tracing taken over a very brief period of time. At times, however, the ECG will reveal an underlying problem such as premature beats, varying degrees of block, conduction defects, a prolonged Q–T interval, Wolff–Parkinson–White syndrome, or other abnormality that may help lead to a diagnosis.[8,9] More often, event monitoring, Holter monitoring, or invasive electrophysiologic testing is needed, especially if the problem is not present at the time of the examination. Rarely, arrhythmias will be more easily seen with exercise testing than with ambulatory monitoring.

The standard ECG is exceptionally useful, however, if it can be obtained during the arrhythmia in question. The 12-lead ECG is an essential tool in making an accurate diagnosis in patients with arrhythmias, as single-lead monitor tracings can be misleading. For an example of this, see Figure 29.

VALVULAR AND CONGENITAL HEART DISEASE

The ECG can be useful in evaluating the effects of valvular heart disease on the myocardium. For example, significant aortic stenosis produces characteristic ECG findings of left ventricular hypertrophy. A number of forms of congenital heart disease produce right ventricular hypertrophy. In addition, there are characteristic ECG findings and patterns which may be quite helpful in the specific diagnosis of congenital heart disease. In general, the ECG is a simple, inexpensive, easily repeated, noninvasive test which may be helpful in qualitatively assessing the effects of congenital or valvular disease or serially following patients over time. However, for good diagnostic accuracy, test such as echocardiography, Doppler, and cardiac catheterization and angiography are more useful.

Thus, while it is important to recognize the limitations of the ECG, it is also one of the most useful, low-risk, inexpensive clinical tools available for diagnosis in patients with heart disease. By using the ECG in an informed way, it is possible to make accurate diagnoses as well as inferences that can be essential in patient management.

5

Abnormalities of Rhythm

INTRODUCTION

The key to reaching the correct diagnosis of an arrhythmia is a systematic approach to the problem—a dissection of the electrocardiogram (ECG) until the relationships become clear. For very complex problems ladder diagrams may be useful but are beyond the scope of this text, as are some of the more unusual rhythm problems. The more common problems in the diagnosis of the cardiac rhythm are discussed here.

Four questions must be answered in order to diagnose the rhythm correctly:

1. Is the rhythm regular or irregular, and is there a pattern to any irregularity seen?
2. What is happening in the ventricles?
3. What is happening in the atria?
4. Then, what is the relationship between the two?

Generally, once these four questions have been answered, the diagnosis will be clear. The process of answering these questions is not, however, always easy. The existence of ectopic beats, unusual waveforms, artifact, different types of block, and differing conduction patterns will at times make the diagnosis of the cardiac rhythm difficult.

Initially, it is easiest to locate the QRS complexes and determine whether they are regular or irregular, and whether there is a pattern to any irregularity seen. In addition, examination of the QRS complexes will help to determine whether the arrhythmia is ventricular or supraventricular. If the QRS complexes are narrow (<0.12 sec) and particularly if the QRS morphology is normal or identical to the QRS morphology previously recorded during normal sinus rhythm, then the rhythm is probably supraventricular, since conduction to the ventricles proceeds over the normal conducting system. If the QRS complexes are wide or different from the QRS complexes during sinus rhythm, then the rhythm usually arises in the ventricles, although it may occasionally be supraventricular, but conducted to the ventricles with "aberration."

In the following discussion, arrhythmias are divided into supraventricular and ventricular arrhythmias, recognizing, of course, that it may not always be possible to easily distinguish between the two. The sections are further subdivided into regular and irregular rhythms.

SUPRAVENTRICULAR ARRHYTHMIAS

Supraventricular arrhythmias are best defined as arrhythmias that arise in or require the participation of structures other than the ventricles. They include, for example, arrhythmias arising in the atria, arising in the atrioventricular (AV) node, or requiring the participation of the atria, AV node, or accessory AV pathways.

To determine what is happening in the atria, one must first search for visible P waves. If none are present, then either atrial standstill or atrial fibrillation may be present. However, there are many times, such as during tachycardias, when atrial activity may be present but not seen because the P waves are buried in the more prominent QRS complexes or the T waves. In these instances, the activity in the atria may have to be inferred from the more evident ventricular response, as noted below. At times there will be what appears to be an occasional P wave or even several in a row during atrial fibrillation. In these cases, the general rule is that if they do not march out in a consistent, regular pattern, then atrial fibrillation is the most likely diagnosis.

If P waves are present, then the next question is "Are the P waves regular or not?" In adults there can be a 10% variation in cycle length as a manifestation of normal sinus rhythm—and the variability can be even greater in children or young adults.

REGULAR SUPRAVENTRICULAR RHYTHMS

Introduction

If P waves are present and regular but there is a rate abnormality, then the atrial rhythm can be categorized as follows:

- *Rate less than 60:* Sinus bradycardia
- *Rate 60–100:* Normal rate
- *Rate 100–250:* Supraventricular tachycardia
  - Normal (e.g., sinus tachycardia)
  - Normal but occurring in setting of other disease process (e.g., sinus tachycardia as a manifestation of fever, congestive heart failure, pulmonary embolus)
  - Abnormal [primary rhythm disturbance, most commonly paroxysmal supraventricular tachycardia (PSVT)]
- *Rate 250–300:* Atrial flutter (rate may be higher or lower in some cases)

Sinus Bradycardia

Bradycardia is frequently a normal finding in well-trained athletes, in persons with healthy hearts, and in persons on beta-blockers. A common cause of abnormal bradycardia is the sick sinus syndrome or bradycardia–tachycardia syndrome, consisting of periods of inappropriately slow atrial activity with or without various supraventricular tachyarrhythmias. It is often not possible on the basis of the ECG tracing alone to state whether the bradycardia is pathological or normal.

Sinus Tachycardia

Sinus tachycardia is usually a normal finding, characterized by a rapid rate originating from the sinus node. A more rapid rate is the normal response of the sinus node to withdrawal of vagal tone or catecholamine stimulation; it occurs normally during exercise, fever, hypotension, and a variety of other normal and abnormal settings. Rarely, sinus tachycardia occurs in isolation without any discernible cause. This is sometimes called "inappropriate" sinus tachycardia and occasionally requires therapy. However, in most cases sinus tachycardia is an appropriate response to a stimulus or condition that calls for a more rapid heart rate.

Atrial Tachycardias

Atrial tachycardias are characterized by regular, rapid atrial activity that originates from areas of the atrium apart from the sinus node. Electrophysiologic studies have suggested that tachycardias that arise from the atrium may be subdivided into automatic atrial tachycardias and sinoatrial or intraatrial reentry tachycardias. Automatic atrial tachycardias are characterized by warmup (a progressive increase of the rate for the few first beats) at the onset of tachycardia. The P waves in automatic atrial tachycardias can be of any configuration. Intraatrial and sinoatrial reentry tachycardias are characterized by paroxysmal onset and offset. Intraatrial reentry can occur anywhere in the atria, and P waves may be of any configuration. Sinoatrial reentry results from reentry in the area surrounding the sinus node, and P waves are similar to those seen in sinus rhythm.[10]

In this sense atrial tachycardias originate solely from atrial tissue and should be distinguished from paroxysmal supraventricular tachycardia (PSVT), previously called paroxysmal atrial tachycardia, or PAT (see below). Carotid massage or other vagal maneuvers that slow AV nodal conduction may create high-grade AV block during atrial tachycardias or atrial flutter and make the P waves more visible and the tachycardia easier to diagnose. However, since the AV node is not required for perpetuation of the tachycardia, vagal maneuvers do not terminate or affect the tachycardia itself, as they will with a PSVT. For a more detailed discussion of these, the reader is referred to the text by Josephson and Seides.[10]

Paroxysmal Supraventricular Tachycardias (Figs. 5 and 6)

This group of dysrhythmias includes tachycardias previously called paroxysmal atrial tachycardia or paroxysmal junctional tachycardia. These rhythms are characterized by abrupt onset, lack of warmup of rate at the onset, and a perfectly regular rhythm. The rate is usually in the range of 140–250 beats/min. The most common electrophysiological mechanism for PSVT is reentry, either within the AV node or AV reentry utilizing an accessory AV pathway. Such accessory pathways either may manifest both antegrade and retrograde conduction (the Wolff–Parkinson–White syndrome) or may be concealed, in which case they conduct only in the retrograde direction.

In AV nodal reentry, there are two pathways within the AV node itself, a slowly conducting and a rapidly conducting pathway. When a premature beat falls at such a time that it conducts exclusively over

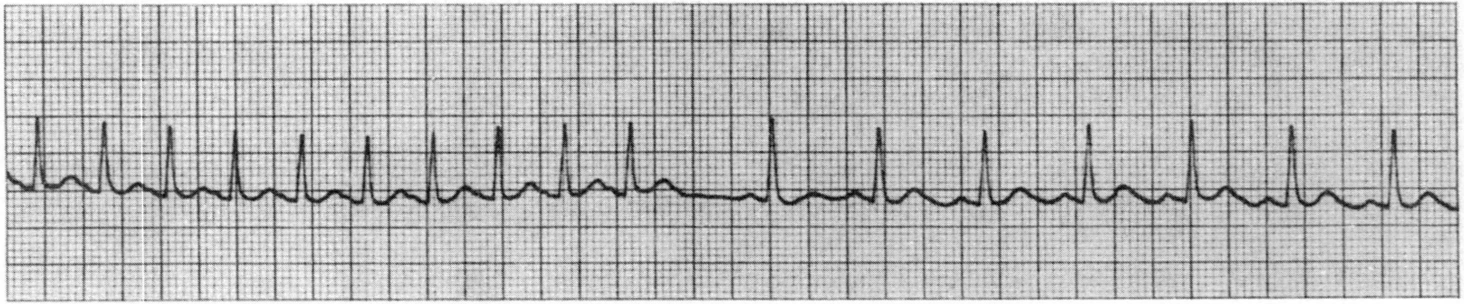

Figure 5. Paroxysmal supraventricular tachycardia. Monitor tracing showing spontaneous termination of the rhythm to a sinus tachycardia. Sudden onset and termination are characteristics of reentrant tachycardias such as this.

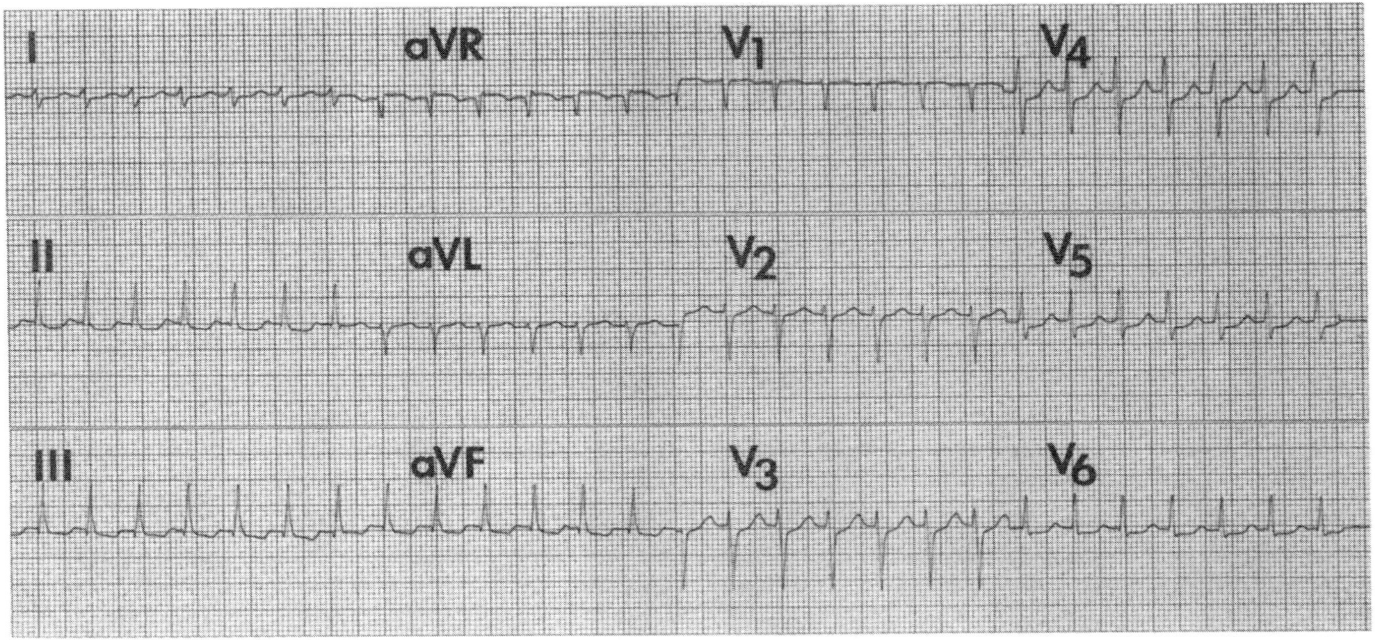

Figure 6. Twelve-lead tracing showing a sustained, regular, narrow-QRS-complex, supraventricular tachycardia (SVT) at 160 beats/min. The QRS duration is normal at 0.08 sec, and the QRS axis and morphology are normal as well, implying that conduction to the ventricles is occurring over the normal conducting system and that this tachycardia is supraventricular. No P waves are visible since they are hidden in the QRS complexes. This patient was shown by electrophysiological study to have SVT due to atrioventricular nodal reentry.

the slow AV nodal pathway, it may then reenter the fast pathway in the retrograde direction and conduct back to the atria, resulting in an atrial echo. If this phenomenon persists, AV nodal reentrant PSVT occurs. Similarly, in patients with an accessory pathway connecting atrium to ventricle, an impulse may conduct exclusively over the normal AV node and His–Purkinje system to the ventricles, then conduct retrograde back to the atria over the accessory pathway, resulting in PSVT. P waves are usually hidden within the QRS complexes in AV nodal reentry and in the ST segment or T waves in reentry utilizing an accessory pathway. The use of vagal maneuvers, such as carotid massage, or activation of the mammalian diving reflex by immersion of the face in cold water may terminate these rhythms by blocking conduction through the AV node. Figures 5 and 6 are ECG tracings showing PSVT.

Rhythms Seen with Wolff–Parkinson–White and Related Syndromes (Fig. 7)

The Wolff–Parkinson–White (WPW) syndrome is characterized by the presence of an accessory pathway connecting atria to ventricles. During normal sinus rhythm, conduction from atria to ventricles occurs over both the normal AV node and His–Purkinje system and over the accessory pathway. Since the accessory pathway behaves electrically much the same as normal ventricular myocardium, it conducts more rapidly and the P–R interval is short and the upstroke of the QRS complex is slurred, giving rise to a delta wave. The QRS complex is thus said to be "preexcited." The remainder of the QRS complex is the result of conduction over the normal conducting system. The presence of a short P–R interval and a delta wave during sinus rhythm due to fusion over both pathways is the hallmark of the WPW syndrome. Patients with the WPW syndrome frequently present with PSVT. In addition, about 30% of patients who present with recurrent PSVT but without manifest WPW syndrome are found at electrophysiologic study to have accessory pathways which are concealed or conduct only in the retrograde direction.

The arrhythmia most commonly associated with the WPW syndrome is regular, narrow-QRS-complex PSVT, due to antegrade conduction to the ventricles over the normal AV node and His–Purkinje system,

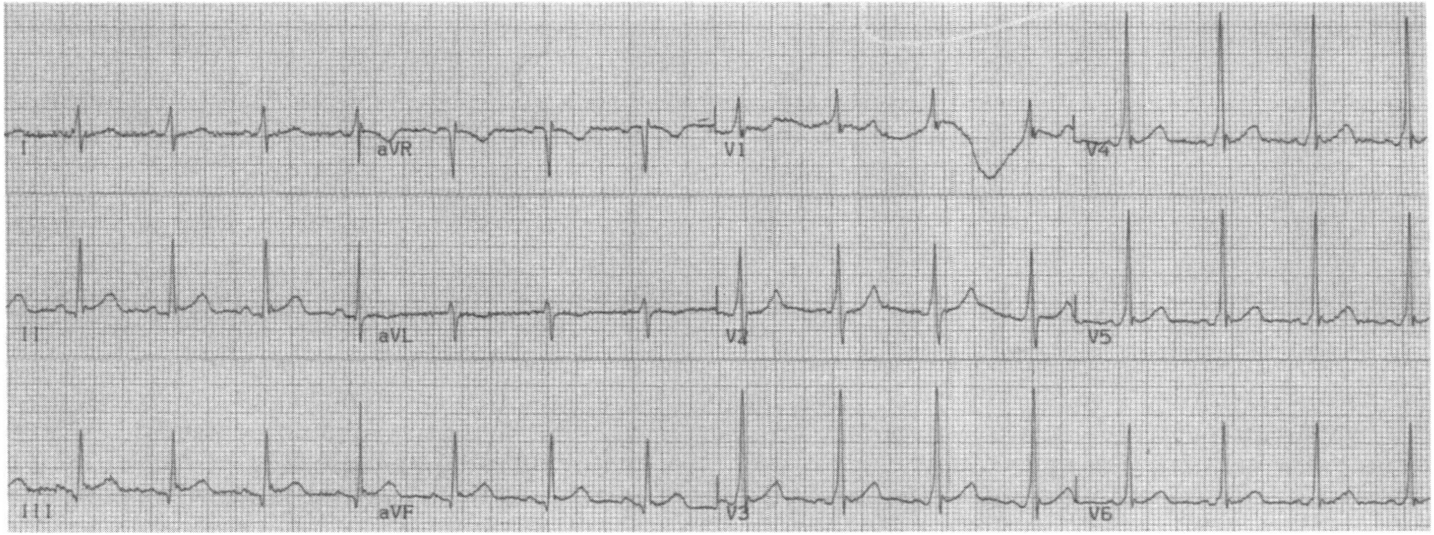

Figure 7. Tracing during normal sinus rhythm showing the findings of Wolff–Parkinson–White syndrome, with a short P–R interval and a delta wave slurring the upstroke of the QRS complexes in the superior and precordial leads. The P–R interval is at the lower limits of normal at 0.10 sec, as seen best in the midprecordium.

followed by retrograde conduction back to the atria over the accessory pathway. This tachycardia is known as orthodromic reciprocating tachycardia. Occasionally, orthodromic tachycardia may be conducted to the ventricles with right bundle branch block or left bundle branch block, resulting in a wide-QRS-complex tachycardia, which is nevertheless supraventricular and is essentially the same in mechanism as the narrow-complex variety.

Less commonly, patients with the WPW syndrome may present with a wide-QRS-complex tachycardia that is quite regular. This antidromic reciprocating tachycardia is due to antegrade conduction over the accessory pathway and retrograde conduction back to the atria over the normal pathway. The QRS complex is thus maximally preexcited and is wide and bizarre.

A more serious arrhythmia associated with the WPW syndrome is atrial fibrillation, which frequently is conducted to the ventricles over the accessory pathway with a very rapid, irregularly irregular ventricular response. This is discussed later under irregular supraventricular arrhythmias.

Atrial Flutter (Figs. 8 and 9)

Classically, atrial flutter is identified by a "sawtooth" pattern of atrial activity most prominent in the inferior leads. The atrial rate is about 300, with the ventricles following at a slower rate. The ventricular rate may be regular if the degree of block is constant or irregular if the degree of AV block is variable. If AV block is constant, it typically occurs in even multiples, i.e., 2:1 or 4:1 block. At times the tracing will alternate between a pattern of atrial flutter and coarse atrial fibrillation. The QRS complexes during atrial flutter may be normal or abnormal, depending on whether or not there is a conduction defect in addition to the expected second-degree AV block. Figures 8 and 9 show atrial flutter.

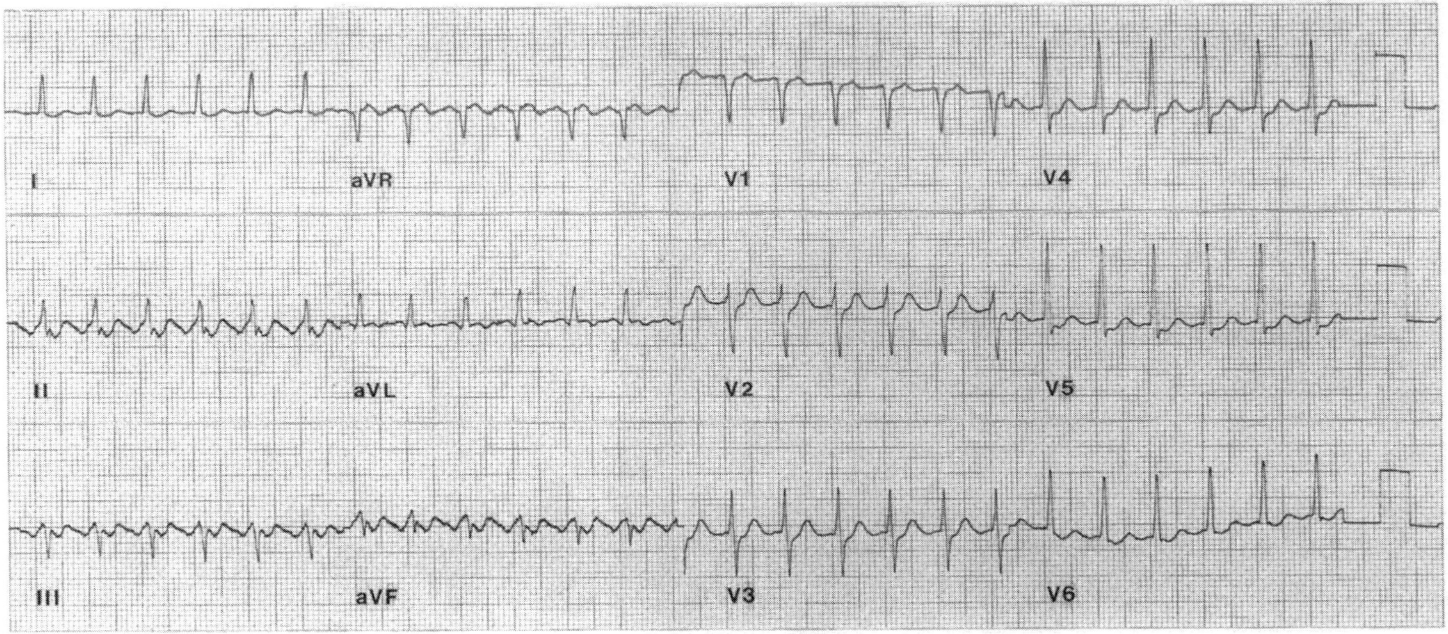

Figure 8. Twelve-lead tracing showing atrial flutter. Note the typical sawtooth appearance in the inferior leads and 2:1 atrioventricular conduction.

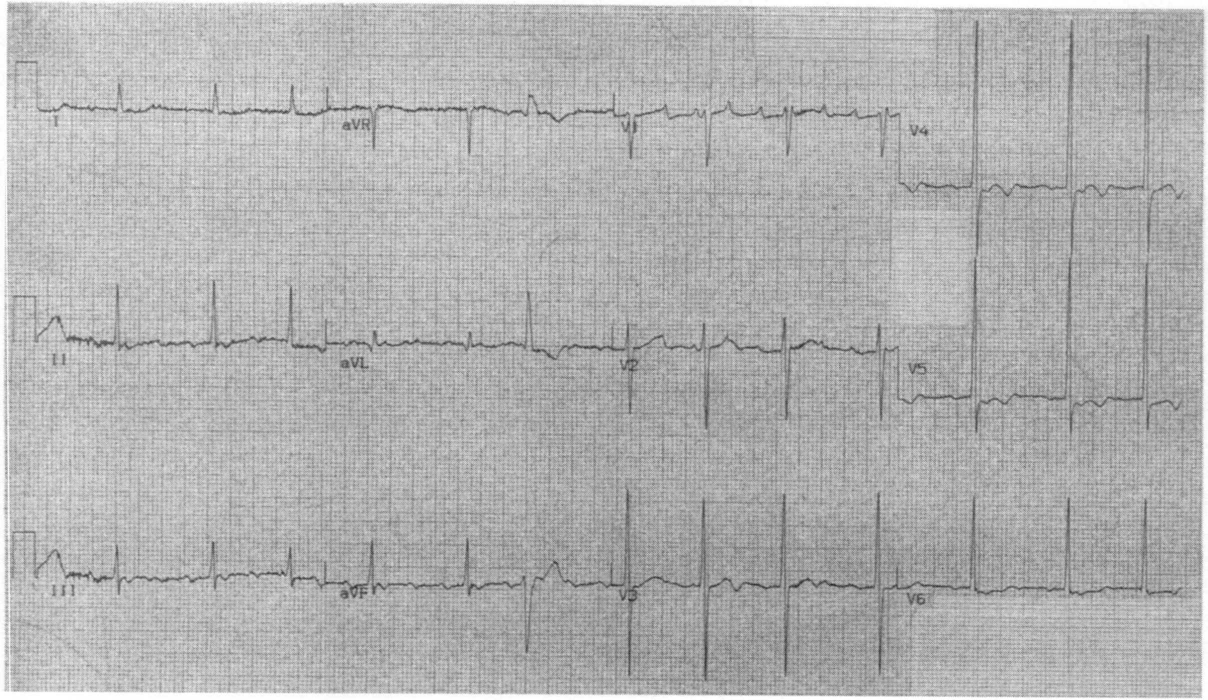

Figure 9. Twelve-lead tracing showing atrial flutter which is less obvious than in Figure 8. The sixth beat is aberrantly conducted. Left ventricular hypertrophy and lateral wall ST–T changes are also present.

Junctional Rhythms (Figs. 10 and 11)

Junctional rhythms are easiest to diagnose when clearly retrograde P waves are present and the QRS complex is normal. Junctional rhythms typically arise in the proximal His–Purkinje system, and direct recording by a catheter placed at the His bundle site shows a His bundle electrogram preceding each QRS

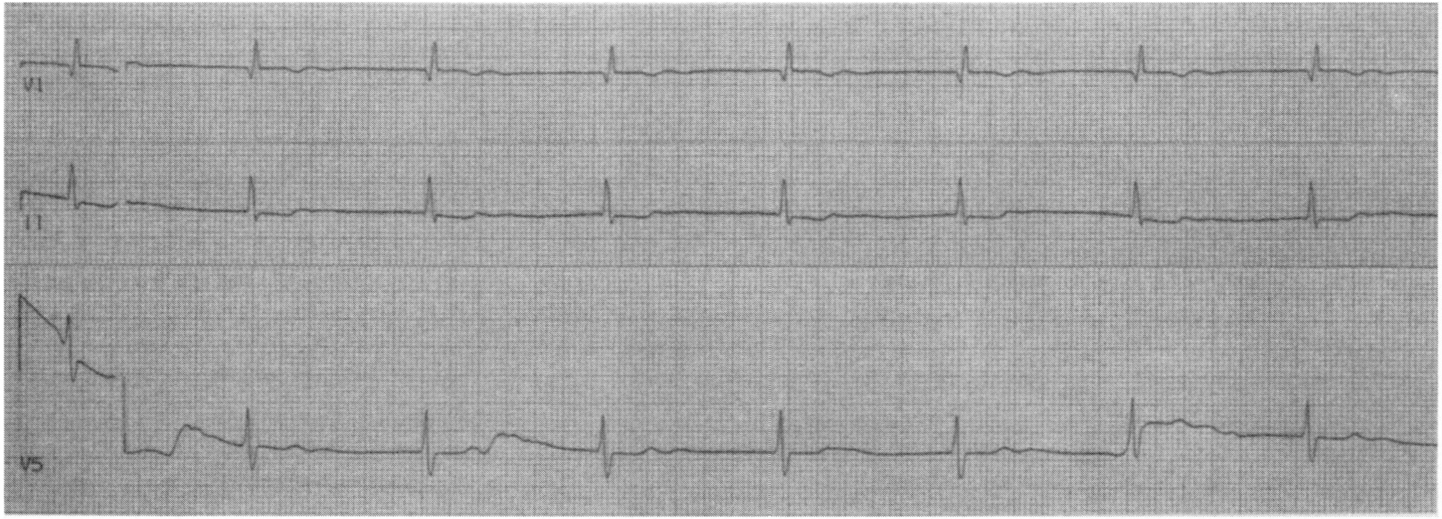

Figure 10. Three-lead rhythm strip showing a junctional rhythm at a rate of 48 beats/min. Either sinus arrest with a junctional escape rhythm, or isorhythmic atrioventricular dissociation could be present. No P waves are seen.

complex. Whether such rhythms ever arise in the AV node itself is controversial. Junctional beats are typically narrow and have a QRS complex identical to that of sinus rhythm, since conduction to the ventricles occurs over the normal conducting system. Junctional beats may be aberrantly conducted, often with an incomplete right bundle branch block (IRBBB) or right bundle branch block (RBBB) pattern, but in the case of wide-QRS-complex rhythms, it is more likely and safer to assume that the rhythm is ventricular in origin rather than junctional.

The ventricular response to a junctional rhythm is usually quite regular, but "capture" beats may cause irregularity if an occasional atrial beat falls at just the right moment to cause an earlier junctional (and ventricular) depolarization (see Fig. 35). If the rate is between 35 and 60, the rhythm is a normal junctional escape rhythm; if between 60 and 100, it is an accelerated junctional rhythm; and if over 100, it is a junctional tachycardia. Junctional escape rhythm occurs when the sinus rate is slow, and the normally slower automatic cells in the AV junction take over the pacemaker function of the heart. Figures 10 and 11 show junctional rhythms.

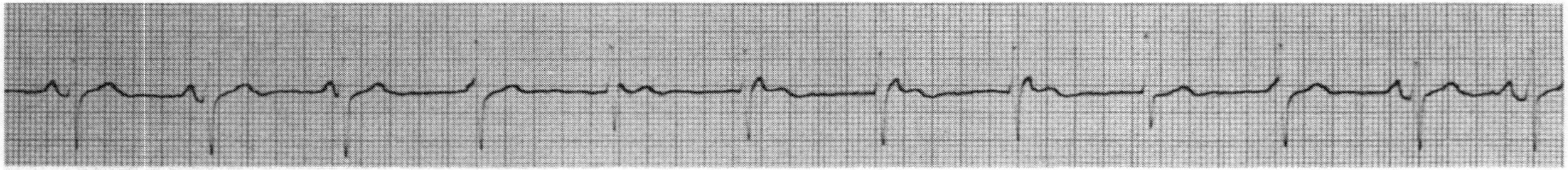

Figure 11. Monitor tracing of an accelerated junctional rhythm with a rate of about 64 beats/min overtaking the sinus rhythm and resulting in atrioventricular dissociation. The last two beats appear to be normally conducted.

IRREGULAR SUPRAVENTRICULAR RHYTHMS

Introduction

If the atrial rate is not regular, then the following diagnoses should be considered:

1. Sinus arrhythmia
2. Premature atrial complexes (PACs)
3. Multifocal atrial rhythm (wandering atrial pacemaker)
4. Multifocal atrial tachycardia
5. Sinus pauses, sinus arrest
6. Junctional complexes with retrograde conduction
7. Ventricular complexes with retrograde conduction
8. Atrial fibrillation (if no consistent P waves are seen)

Sinus Arrhythmia

Sinus arrhythmia is normal if the beat-to-beat variation in cycle length is 10% or less. Sinus arrhythmia occurs as a result of respiratory-linked oscillations in vagal tone and is greater in young patients or patients with a high level of resting vagal tone. All P waves should be identical, upright in lead II, and the P–R intervals should be constant.

Premature Atrial Complexes (Figs. 12–14)

PACs are characterized by early P waves, often with a different configuration and different PR interval. They may occur in isolation or can occur at some fixed ratio to the normal P waves, giving rise to atrial bigeminy, trigeminy, or similar rhythm. PACs can at times be difficult to differentiate from premature junctional contractions. This is because the retrograde P wave resulting from the junctional discharge may occur prior to the QRS complex, suggesting an atrial origin for the impulse. PACs are frequently seen in normal individuals, but can also occur with a variety of cardiac diseases. In the setting of serious illness, including myocardial infarction, they may be an early sign of atrial overload and congestive heart failure.

Usually, a PAC will reset the sinus node pacemaker and advance the timing of the next sinus beat. The next P wave is often slightly delayed, however, from the timing that would be expected if the PAC instantly reset the sinus node pacemaker with no other alteration in rhythm. This occurs because the impulse must be conducted to the area of the sinus node and into the sinus node itself before the rhythm of the sinus node is reset. At the time of the next sinus impulse, the depolarization wave must likewise exit from the sinus node to the atrium before the next P wave is inscribed on the ECG. Thus, when a PAC resets the sinus node, the interval from the PAC until the next sinus beat is equal to the sinus cycle length plus the conduction time into and back out of the sinus node (the sinoatrial conduction time).

It is possible that the delay will cause the postpremature beat to occur at the end of a pause that

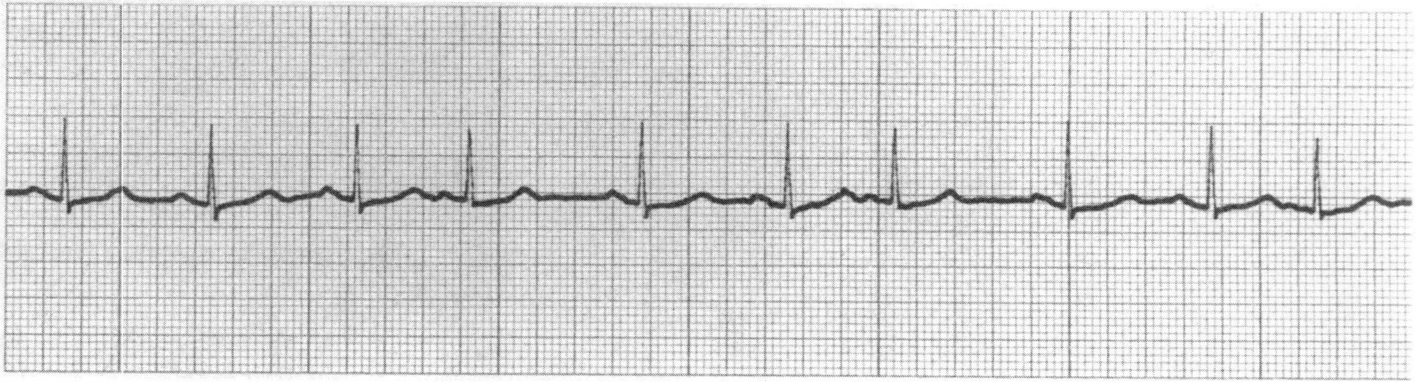

Figure 12. Tracing showing isolated atrial premature (fourth, seventh, and tenth) beats.

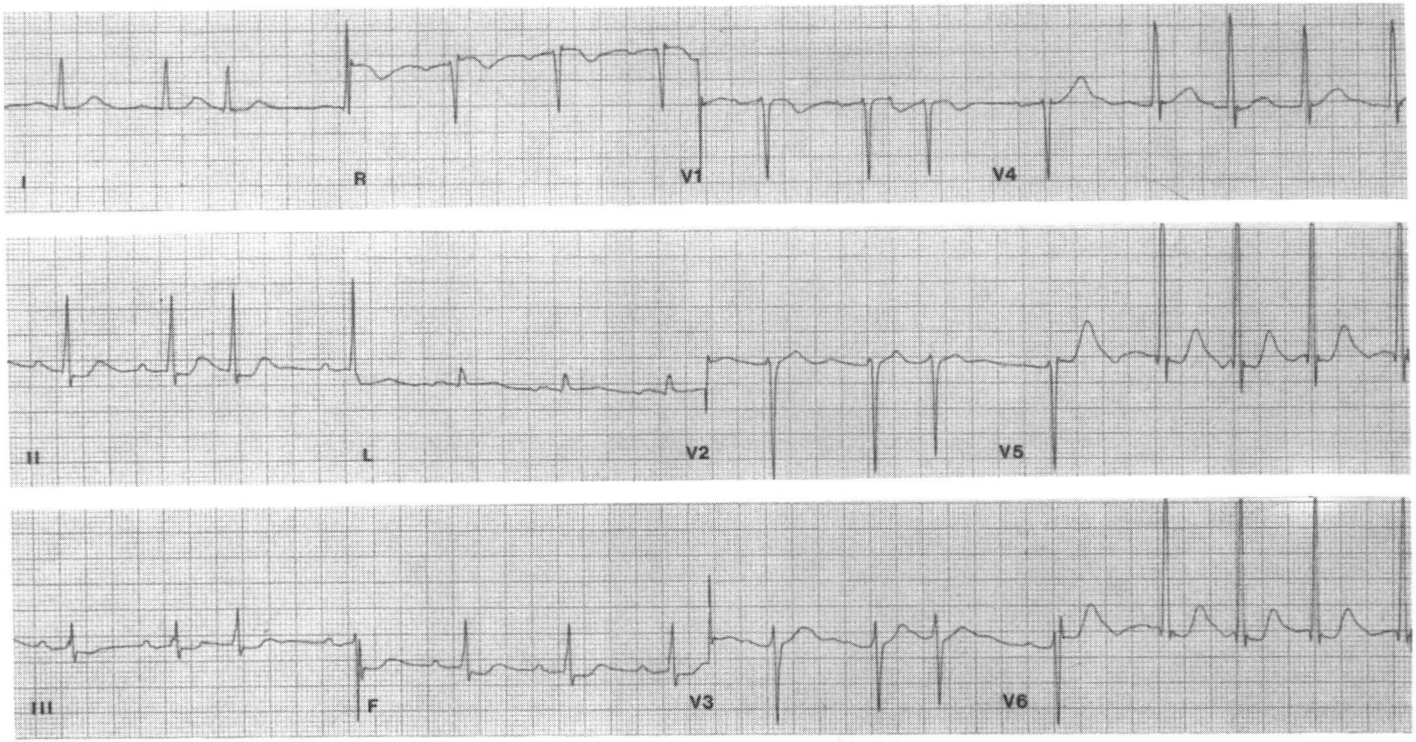

Figure 13. Twelve-lead tracing showing PACs with hard-to-find premature P waves, which are nearly hidden in the preceding T Wave. Left ventricular hypertrophy, with inferior and lateral ST segment depression suggestive of strain or ischemia, is also present.

is almost exactly compensatory. If, in addition, the PAC is conducted aberrantly resulting in an abnormal QRS, it may be difficult to distinguish the PAC from a PVC. This is especially true if the P wave is hidden under the T wave of the preceding complex. Figures 12–14 show PACs. Figure 13 shows PACs with the premature P waves nearly hidden in the T wave of the preceding complex, and Figure 14 shows a PAC conducted with typical aberration.

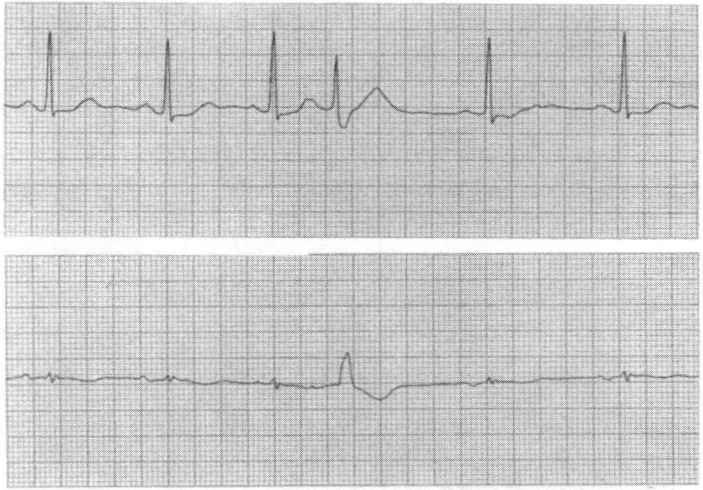

Figure 14. In this tracing the fourth beat is an atrial premature beat which is conducted to the ventricles with right bundle branch block or aberration. The atrial origin of this beat is apparent because the P wave can be seen superimposed on the previous T wave. The impulse arrives at the His–Purkinje system at a time when the right bundle branch is still refractory, but the left bundle branch has recovered and is able to conduct, hence the appearance of right bundle branch block.

Wandering Atrial Pacemaker (Multifocal Atrial Rhythm) (Fig. 15)

Wandering atrial pacemaker may occur in normal individuals, especially those with a high level of vagal tone. There may be several types of P waves distinguished by morphology and/or P–R intervals, and the rate is less than 100 by definition. The rhythm may alternate irregularly between atrial and junctional origins. It may also be associated with a variety of cardiac diseases including rheumatic fever. An example of wandering atrial pacemaker is shown in Figure 15.

Multifocal Atrial Tachycardia (Fig. 16)

Multifocal atrial tachycardia has a rate of over 100, with at least three different P-wave morphologies and/or P–R intervals. It can at times be difficult to distinguish from atrial fibrillation if the atrial activity is so chaotic that clear repetitive P-wave activity is not immediately evident. Patients with this rhythm have a high mortality, not because of the rhythm *per se* but rather because of the serious nature of the illnesses with which it is associated (generally severe pulmonary disease).

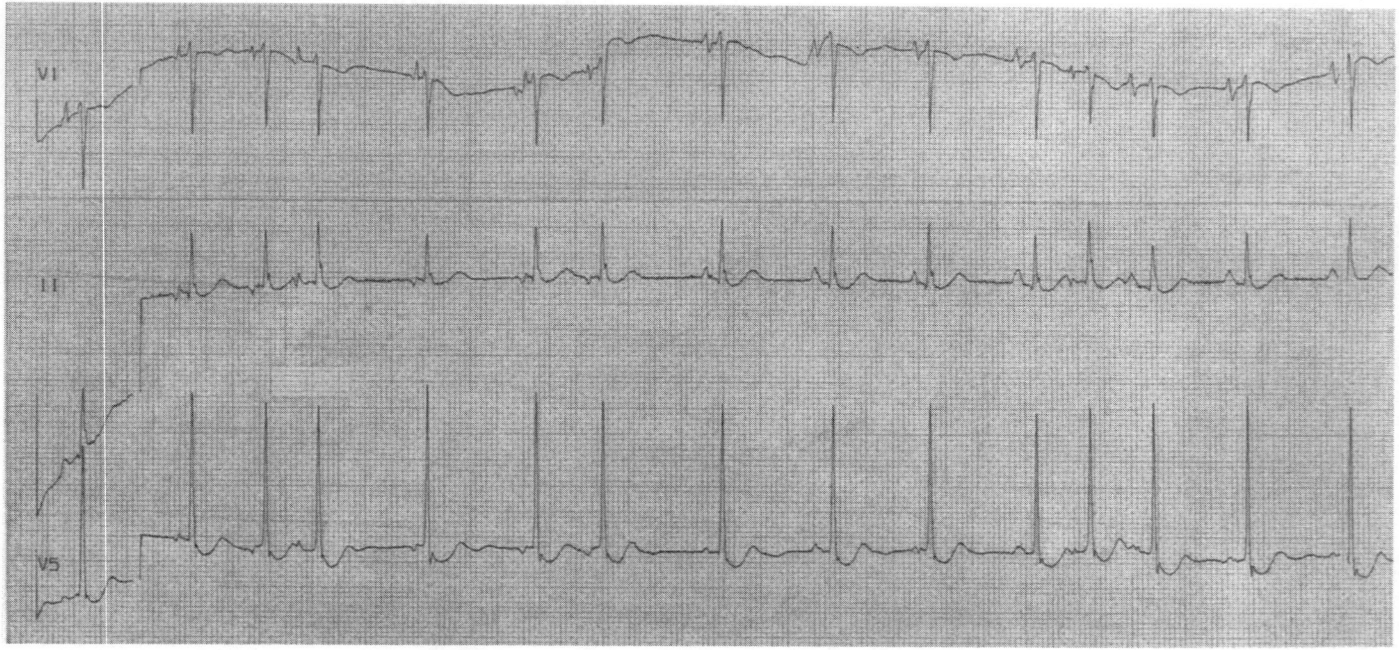

Figure 15. This three-lead rhythm strip shows at least three distinct P-wave morphologies and a rate varying between 70 and 150, which is characteristic of a wandering atrial pacemaker.

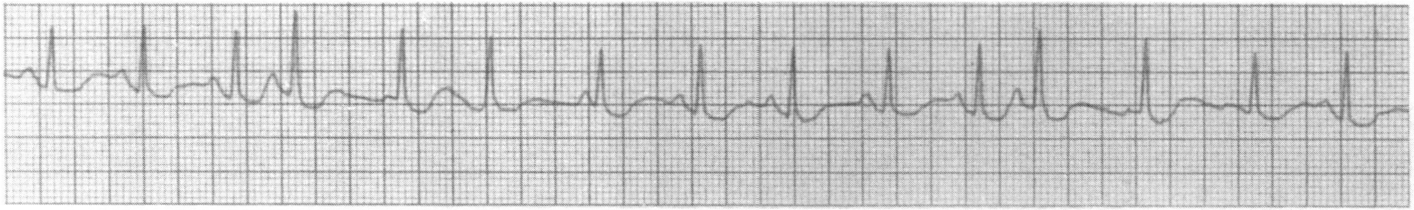

Figure 16. Tracing showing multifocal atrial tachycardia, with several different P-wave morphologies and P–R intervals, in a patient with severe chronic obstructive pulmonary disease.

Sinus Pauses and Sinus Arrest (Figs. 17 and 18)

In these rhythms, atrial activity simply ceases for a period of time. Normally a lower pacemaker in the AV junction or the ventricle eventually escapes at a lower rate and takes over the normal pacemaker function of the heart. However, the lower pacemakers may not be reliable and sinus arrest may result in long periods of asystole and loss of consciousness.

The sinoatrial node is subject to other types of rhythm abnormalities. Figure 18 shows grouped P waves, probably resulting from Wenckebach-type SA node exit block.

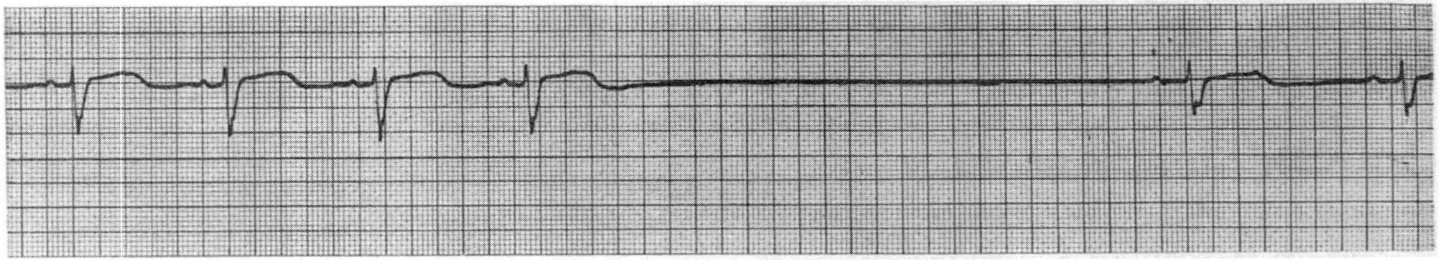

Figure 17. This monitor strip shows an episode of spontaneous sinus arrest lasting 5 sec.

Premature Junctional Complexes

See previous discussion. Premature junctional complexes (PJCs) may give rise to P waves by retrograde conduction to the atria. Usually these retrograde P waves will reset the sinus node pacemaker, giving rise to atrial irregularities. Retrograde atrial activation due to PJCs can be manifested by P waves that can occur before, after, or during the QRS complex.

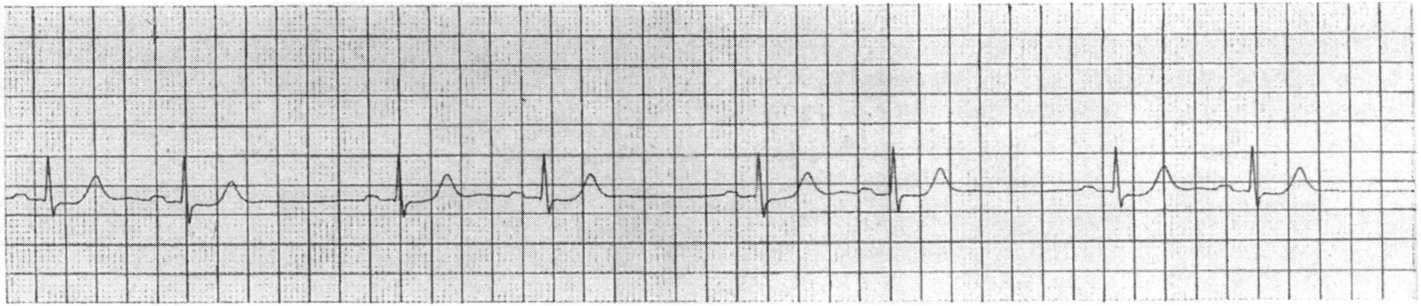

Figure 18. Grouped P waves in this tracing suggest sinoatrial (SA) nodal exit block, probably sinoatrial Wenckebach.

Atrial Fibrillation (Fig. 19)

In atrial fibrillation the atria are continually being depolarized by shifting wave fronts of activation at rates up to 600/min. This disorganized atrial activity may be seen as fine fibrillatory waves on the ECG between QRS complexes or may not be apparent at all if the amplitude is too low. The ventricles are protected from being activated at such rapid rates by the phenomenon of concealed conduction, which keeps the AV node in a partially refractory state.

The rate of the ventricular response during atrial fibrillation varies depending on the ability of the AV node to conduct impulses. The ventricular response is classically irregularly irregular because of the constantly varying degree of concealed conduction into the AV node. The phenomenon of concealed conduction in atrial fibrillation accounts for the fact that control of the ventricular rate is generally easier when the rhythm is atrial fibrillation than when it is atrial flutter. With atrial flutter the bombardment of the AV node by atrial impulses is slower than it is with atrial fibrillation and thus the AV node is in a less refractory state, thereby making more rapid ventricular rates common with atrial flutter.

Because of the differing cycle lengths in atrial fibrillation, it is not uncommon for the ventricular complexes to have different morphologies which can give the appearance of PVCs. This is especially likely if there are conduction disturbances such as rate-dependent bundle branch block. The Ashman phenomenon (discussed in the next section) is sometimes the cause of wide-QRS-complex beats occurring during atrial fibrillation. Figure 19 shows atrial fibrillation occurring in a patient with preexisting left bundle branch block (LBBB) pattern. Note how this could easily be mistaken, especially on a monitor tracing, for a slow ventricular tachycardia were it not for the grossly irregular rate.

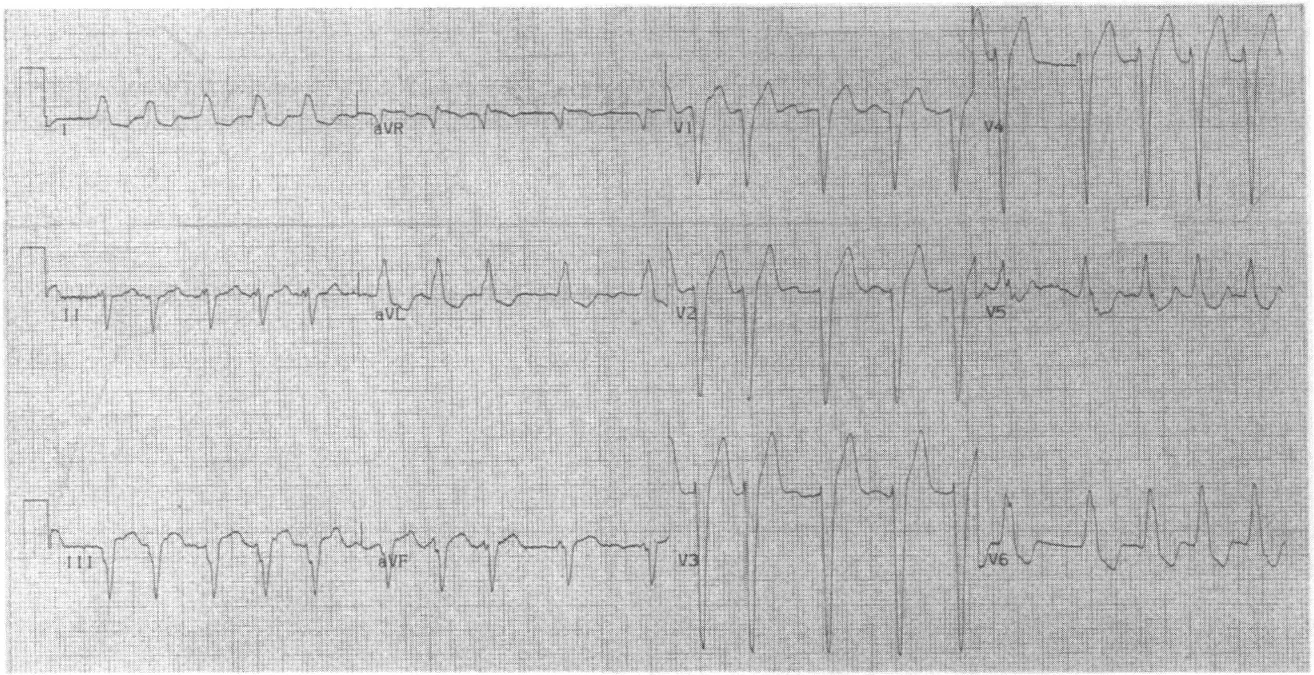

Figure 19. This twelve-lead tracing shows atrial fibrillation occurring in a patient with LBBB. The rate is not well controlled. The patient was 101 years old when the tracing was taken.

Irregularity and the Ashman Phenomenon (Fig. 20)

The Ashman phenomenon is the tendency for aberrant conduction to occur when a short R–R interval follows a longer one despite the fact that conduction in a string of shorter R–R intervals may be normal. This occurs because the longer R–R interval results in a longer repolarization phase and thus a longer refractory period. If conduction down one of the pathways is marginal, then the impulse following the shorter R–R interval may enter the conducting pathway during a time when part of the conducting system is still refractory. Thus, the beat following the short R–R interval will be conducted aberrantly.

The aberrant conduction pattern may be in the form of bundle branch block, most commonly RBBB, and it may be rate dependent, occurring whenever the R–R interval becomes sufficiently short. These considerations are most useful in the setting of atrial fibrillation when some abnormal ventricular complexes are seen, and the question arises as to whether they represent PVCs or aberrantly conducted supraventricular impulses. Figure 20 shows an aberrantly conducted beat demonstrating the Ashman phenomenon.

Atrial Fibrillation in Patients with WPW

As mentioned earlier, patients with the WPW syndrome are particularly prone to the development of atrial fibrillation, which is often conducted to the ventricles over both the normal pathway (AV node and His–Purkinje system) and the accessory pathway. Since the accessory pathway lacks the normal filtering capacity of the AV node, which limits the rate at which impulses can be conducted to the ventricles, atrial fibrillation may be conducted over the accessory pathway with ventricular rates as high as 300 beats/min. This tachycardia is characterized by an irregularly irregular rhythm and QRS complexes that are wide but may vary from narrow to wide owing to varying degrees of fusion of atrial fibrillation over the normal and accessory pathways.

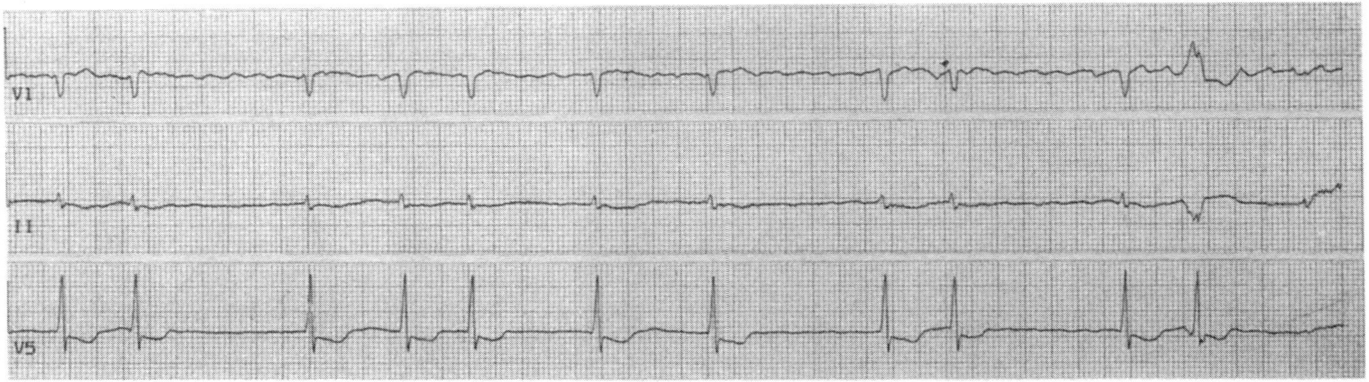

Figure 20. This three-lead rhythm strip shows atrial fibrillation with the final complex demonstrating the Ashman phenomenon. Interestingly, the preceding pair of complexes, which has almost exactly the same R–R interval, does not show aberrant conduction. The importance of multiple leads is well demonstrated by this tracing—if one were to look just at lead 2, this lead would appear to be most likely ventricular in origin, and if one looked at V5, the abnormality of conduction could be missed altogether.

REGULAR VENTRICULAR RHYTHMS

Introduction

Rhythms that arise in the ventricles and have regular ventricular complexes fall into the following categories:

1. Ventricular escape rhythm
2. Accelerated idioventricular rhythm
3. Ventricular tachycardia
4. Ventricular paced rhythms

Ventricular Escape Rhythm (Fig. 21)

A ventricular escape rhythm may occur when the normal higher pacemakers in the heart, typically the sinus node and AV junction, default and fail to maintain an adequate rate. At rates of around 40 and below, Purkinje cells and even ventricular myocardial cells are capable of behaving in an automatic fashion, and they take over the normal pacemaker function of the heart. This results in a slow, wide-QRS-complex ventricular escape rhythm. Figure 21 provides an example of a ventricular escape rhythm, as does Figure 42.

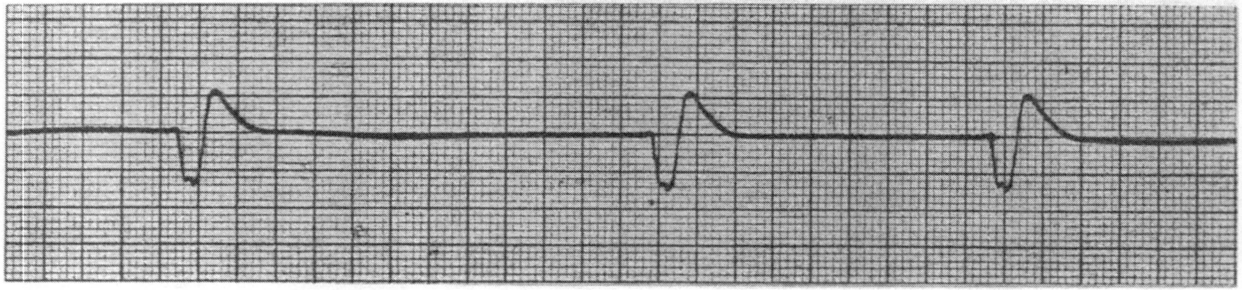

Figure 21. No atrial activity is seen. The rhythm is a slow, wide-complex, ventricular escape rhythm.

Accelerated Idioventricular Rhythm (Fig. 22)

This rhythm arises in the ventricle and is distinguished from ventricular tachycardia primarily by its rate. This arrhythmia has a rate of less than 100 beats/min, is characterized by wide QRS complexes, and is usually nonsustained (lasting less than 30 sec). Because of the slow rate, atrial activity in the form of dissociated P waves or ventricular fusion beats are commonly seen. This rhythm disorder is commonly seen in the setting of acute myocardial infarction. Figure 22 shows a brief run of accelerated idioventricular rhythm.

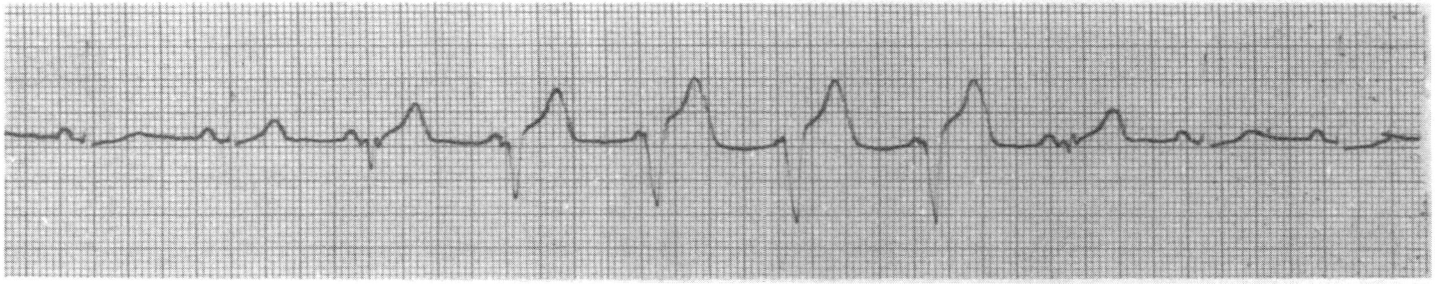

Figure 22. An accelerated ventricular rhythm with a rate of about 75 overtakes a slightly slower sinus rate. Atrioventricular dissociation is present, and the third, fourth, and eighth complexes are clearly fusion beats, proving the ventricular origin of the abnormal complexes.

Ventricular Tachycardia (Figs. 23–26)

Ventricular tachycardia is a serious rhythm disorder characterized by a rate greater than 100 beats/min. Rates of much greater than 200 beats/min are less commonly seen in clinical settings, probably because at more rapid rates there is a higher incidence of degeneration to ventricular fibrillation. However, despite the serious and life-threatening nature of this arrhythmia, patients may present in a relatively stable hemodynamic state with sustained ventricular tachycardia, particularly when the rate is slow. The ECG typically shows a wide (>0.12 sec) QRS complex, and the rhythm is usually regular. The QRS morphology varies depending on the site in the ventricles from which the tachycardia arises. At more rapid rates, it may be difficult to distinguish the QRS complex from the ST segment and T wave, and the rhythm appears sinusoidal. Ventricular tachycardia is most common in patients with structural heart disease, most often coronary artery disease or cardiomyopathy, although it may occur in patients with other forms of heart disease or without any organic heart disease.

P waves may sometimes be seen during the tachycardia if they are not obscured by the wide, bizarre QRS complexes. If there is intact retrograde conduction, there may be a 1:1 relationship between QRS complexes and P waves, despite the fact that the atria are not involved in the tachycardia itself, but are merely being activated passively. More commonly, there is complete dissociation between atrial and ventricular activity. In this case, careful observation may sometimes disclose either evidence of dissociated P-wave activity on the ECG or the presence of capture beats. The latter are caused by the conduction of an occasional P wave to the ventricles over the normal conducting system, resulting in a normal, narrow QRS complex. The presence of fusion beats, caused by fusion between such conducted P waves and the ventricular tachycardia beats, proves a ventricular origin of the rhythm. Figures 36 and 37 show examples of ventricular capture and fusion.

Differentiation between ventricular tachycardia and supraventricular tachycardia with aberrancy may be difficult. This issue is discussed in more detail later. However, sustained wide-QRS-complex tachycardias are much more likely to be ventricular in origin rather than supraventricular, and it is safer

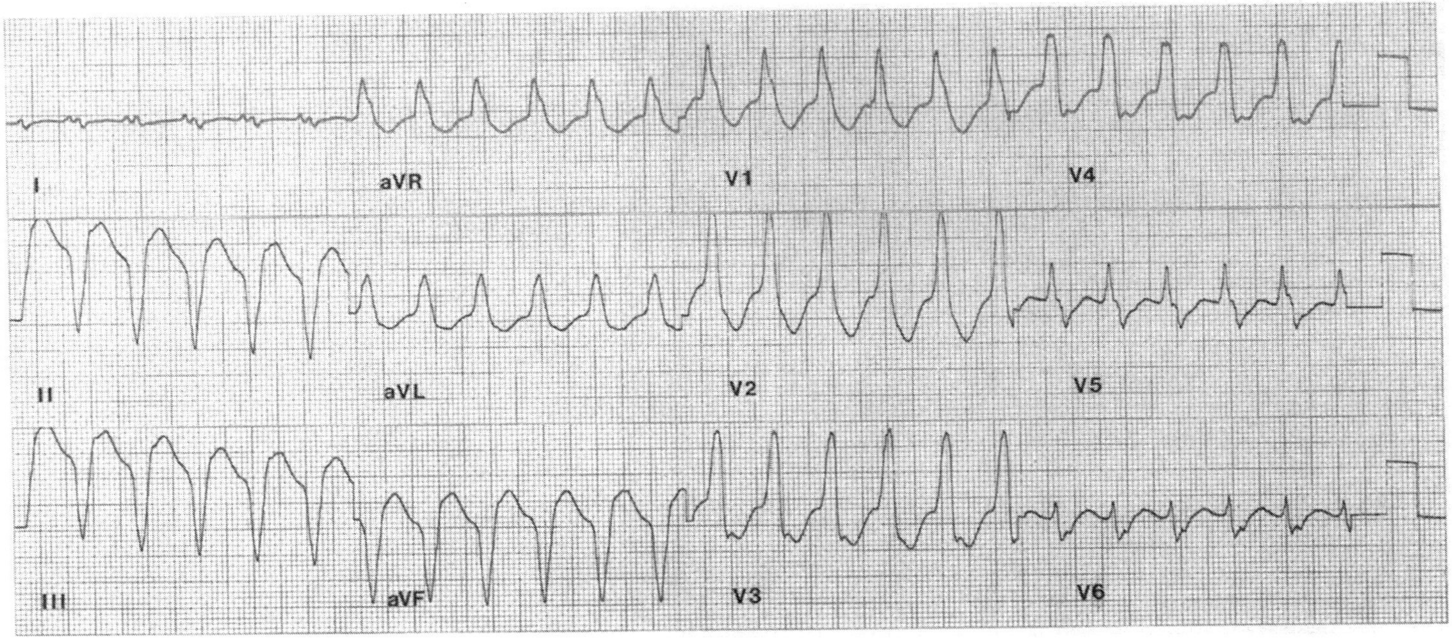

Figure 23. Twelve-lead electrocardiogram showing sustained ventricular tachycardia.

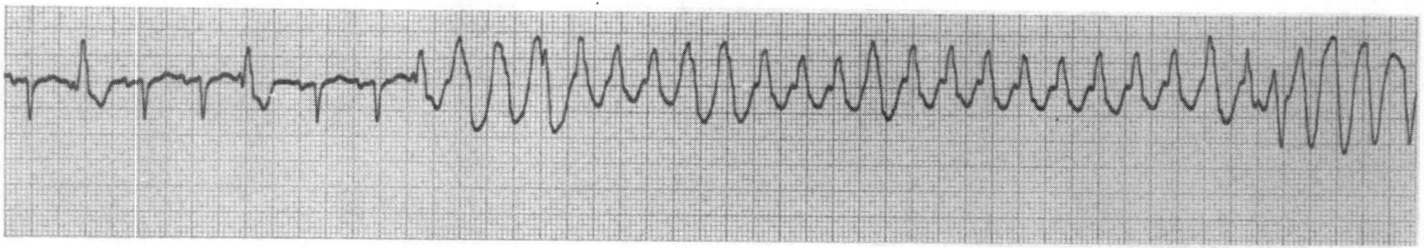

Figure 24. Polymorphic ventricular tachycardia.

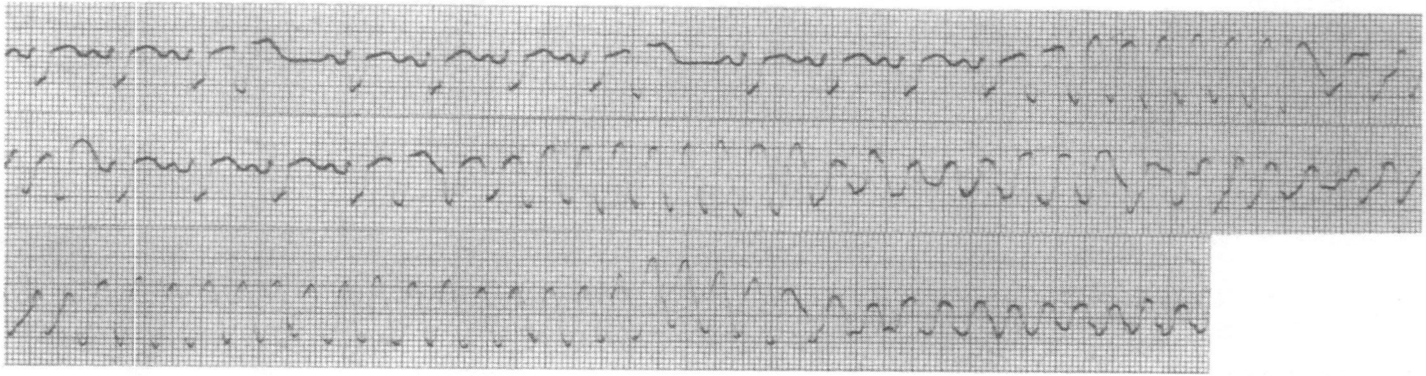

Figure 25. Continuous-monitor tracing of two runs of ventricular tachycardia, the second of which appears to degenerate. There was a conduction disturbance, most likely left bundle branch block, prior to the ventricular tachycardia.

clinically to assume, when in doubt, that such arrhythmias are ventricular tachycardia and to treat them as such. This is especially true when there is a high likelihood of coronary artery disease. Figures 23–25 show examples of common forms of ventricular tachycardia.

Repetitive monomorphic ventricular tachycardia is a variety of ventricular tachycardia seen occasionally in patients who are most often free of structural heart disease. This entity is characterized by multiple short runs of ventricular tachycardia separated by varying periods of sinus rhythm. There may be so many runs that the ventricular tachycardia predominates, and the ventricular beats tend to be all of one morphology. The prognosis in this disorder is generally good, and many such patients do not appear to require any antiarrhythmic drug therapy.[11] Figure 26 is a rhythm strip from a patient with repetitive monomorphic ventricular tachycardia.

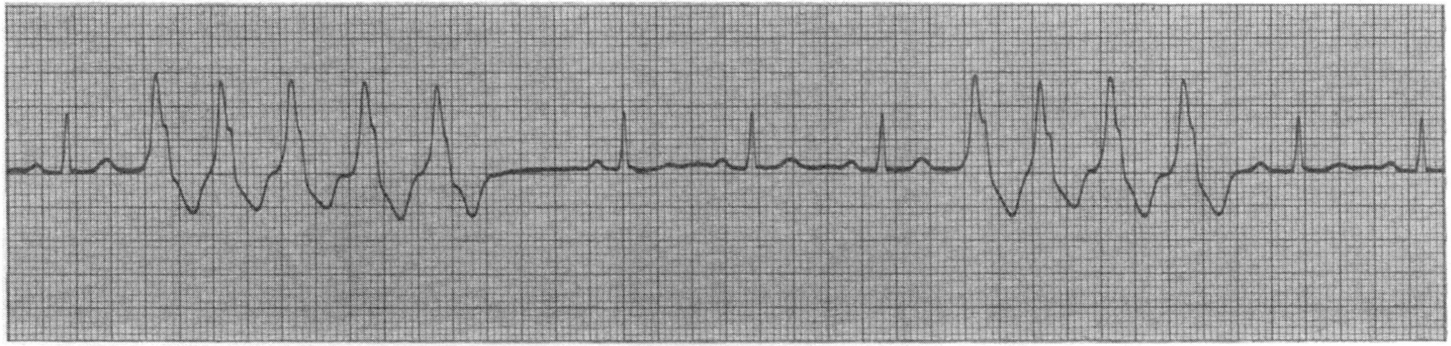

Figure 26. Rhythm strip from a patient with repetitive monomorphic ventricular tachycardia.

Paced Rhythms (Fig. 27)

Ventricular pacing is a common cause of a regular, wide-QRS-complex rhythm. Usually, a sharp pacemaker stimulus artifact ("pacer spike") appears before each QRS complex, but the presence of a pacemaker artifact may be overlooked, especially if the quality of the tracing is less than excellent. Clues include a wide QRS with a LBBB pattern and left-axis deviation (since most ventricular pacing is from the right ventricular apex) and in most cases absolute regularity of the paced beats. AV dissociation is seen if unpaced atrial activity is present. Figure 27 is an example of a tracing with a dual-chamber pacemaker. Figure 34 shows a rhythm with paced and nonpaced beats with pacemaker fusion beats. Ventricular pacing is not always at a fixed rate, however. Dual-chamber pacemakers are designed, among other modes, to sense atrial activity and pace the ventricle after a fixed AV interval. Thus, they can exhibit ventricular pacing at a rate as irregular as the sensed atrial rate that drives it. Other variable-rate pacemakers are capable of pacing at variable ventricular rates in response to the perceived need for an increase or decrease in rate based on activity, temperature, or other parameters.

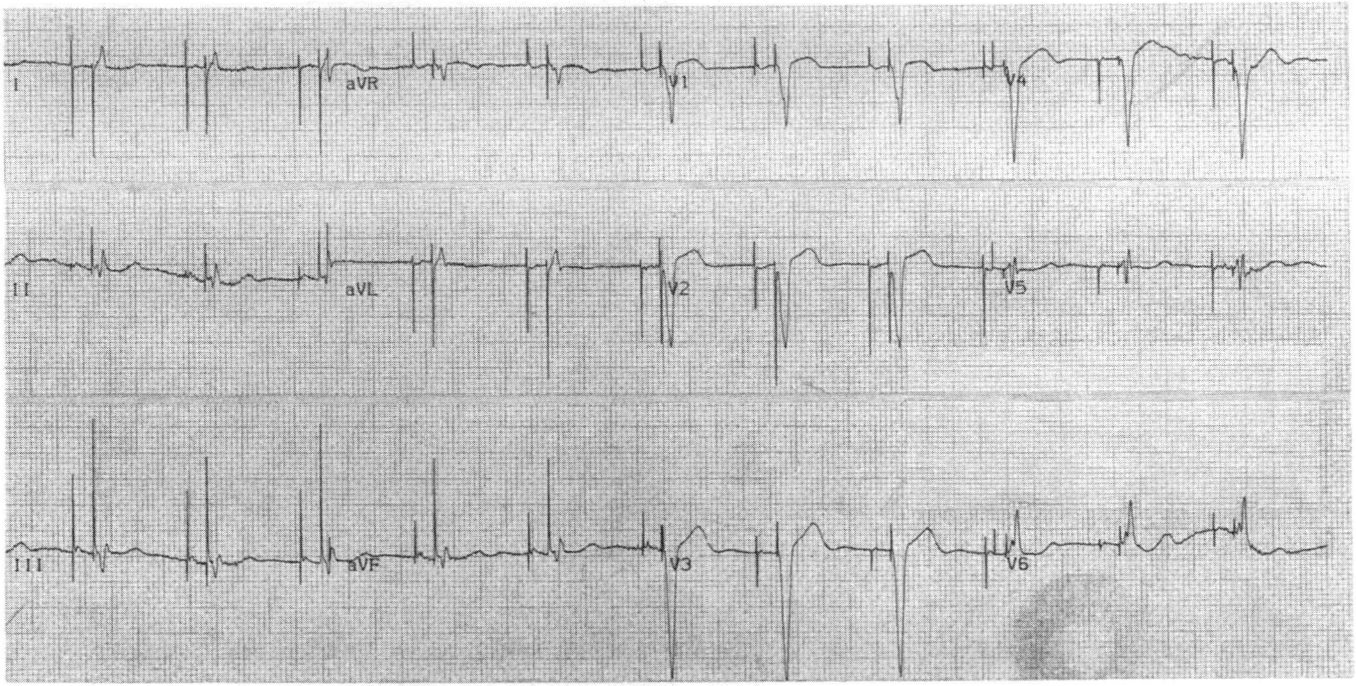

Figure 27. This twelve-lead tracing shows dual-chamber pacing.

IRREGULAR VENTRICULAR RHYTHMS

Introduction

The rhythms with irregular ventricular activity fall into the following categories:

1. Premature ventricular complexes (PVCs)
2. *Torsade de pointes*
3. Ventricular fibrillation
4. Irregular ventricular paced rhythms, or rhythms that are a mixture of paced and unpaced rhythm
5. Capture beats interrupting a regular ventricular rhythm
6. Ventricular complexes that are irregular because of block or interference effects on the transmission of a supraventricular rhythm (e.g., atrial tachycardia or flutter with block, Mobitz I and Mobitz II blocks)

Premature Ventricular Complexes (Figs. 28–31)

The PVC is perhaps the most common rhythm disturbance and occurs from time to time in most healthy people as well as in patients with heart disease. The hallmark is a premature QRS complex which is wide and bizarre and which usually has a T-wave vector opposite the QRS vector. A variety of names have been used, including premature ventricular complexes or contractions and ventricular premature beats or depolarizations. Identification of the abnormal-looking QRS complex is not difficult. However, it is sometimes difficult to distinguish a premature beat of ventricular origin from a supraventricular premature beat that is conducted to the ventricles with aberrancy. In addition, PVCs can sometimes have narrow QRS complexes and can mimic supraventricular beats, particularly if only one ECG lead is available for analysis. Most often the PVC does not interrupt the normal sinus rhythm and thus

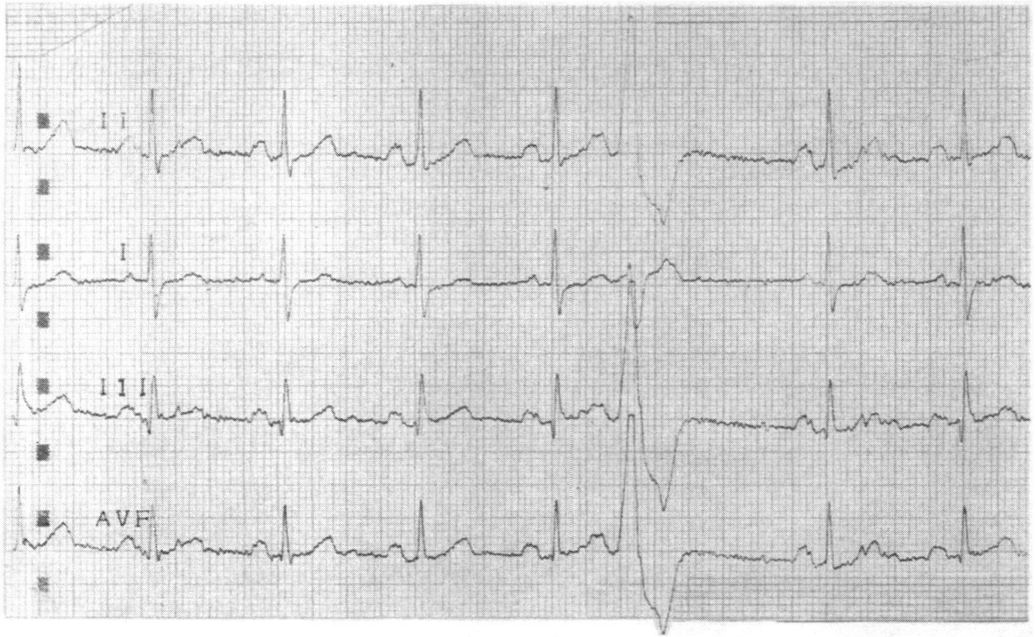

Figure 28. A premature ventricular complex. The atrial pacemaker is not reset and the pause following the PVC is compensatory.

the pause after the PVC is "fully compensatory"; i.e., the interval between the two normal beats before and after the PVC is exactly equal to two normal R–R intervals. However, PVCs may also be interpolated and thus not disturb the normal sinus mechanism at all, or they may conduct back to the atria and reset the sinus node. (See Fig. 28.)

A 12-lead ECG, or at least a multilead monitor tracing, is often necessary to determine whether a premature beat (or tachycardia) is supraventricular with aberrant conduction or ventricular in origin, as ventricular beats may masquerade as supraventricular beats. Figure 29 illustrates how confusion may occur.

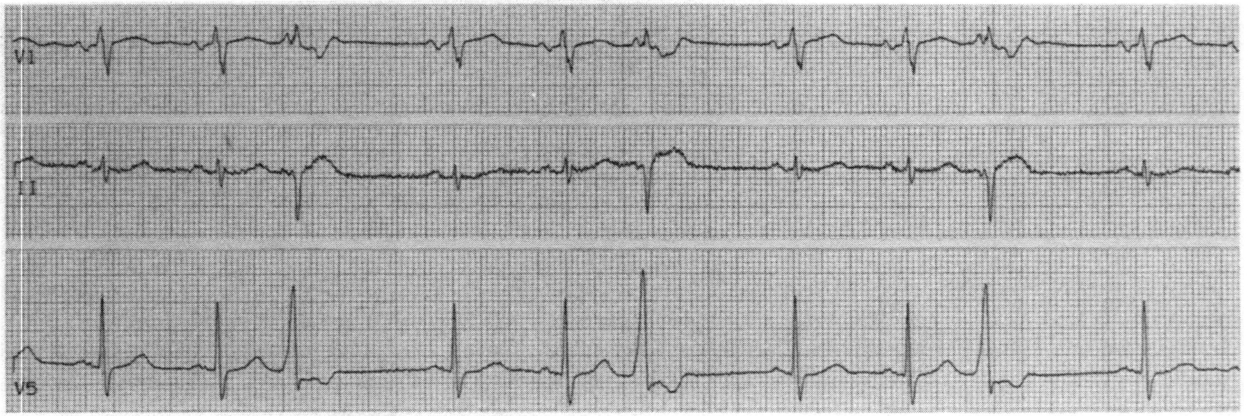

Figure 29. PVCs. Note that the premature complexes in V1 have a configuration that resembles a premature P wave preceding each QRS complex. This suggests the possibility of PACs with aberrant conduction to the ventricles. However, the P–R intervals in this tracing are too short to be conducted. Study of the other two simultaneous leads shows that the first deflection is actually part of the QRS complex and is thus not a P wave at all.

Thus, the presence of dissociated atrial activity, a compensatory pause after the PVC, and certain morphological criteria are sometimes helpful in diagnosing premature beats as ventricular, but no such criteria can be used to distinguish between ventricular and supraventricular premature beats with certainty. When in doubt, it is safest clinically to assume that wide-QRS-complex beats are ventricular in origin until proven otherwise.

The presence of the Ashman phenomenon, the consistent occurrence of the abnormal complex following a long–short pattern of R–R intervals, suggests that the complex in question may be supraventricular in origin. This is most often seen during atrial fibrillation. (See text and Fig. 20.)

Similarly, if the occurrence of an abnormal beat is clearly rate dependent (that is, the abnormality occurs when the sinus rate reaches a critical level), it may be a supraventricular beat with aberrant conduction. The diagnosis here is usually assisted by the continuing presence of P waves related to the QRS complexes. However, other ventricular dysrhythmias can be rate dependent as well. Examples of this are seen in Figures 30 and 31, which show rate-dependent LBBBs.

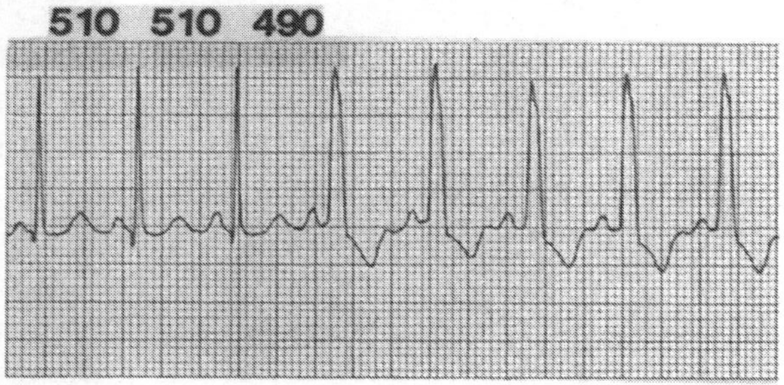

Figure 30. Rate-dependent left bundle branch block with the change in conduction occurring when the rate exceeds 120. Intervals between beats (msec) are shown above the tracing.

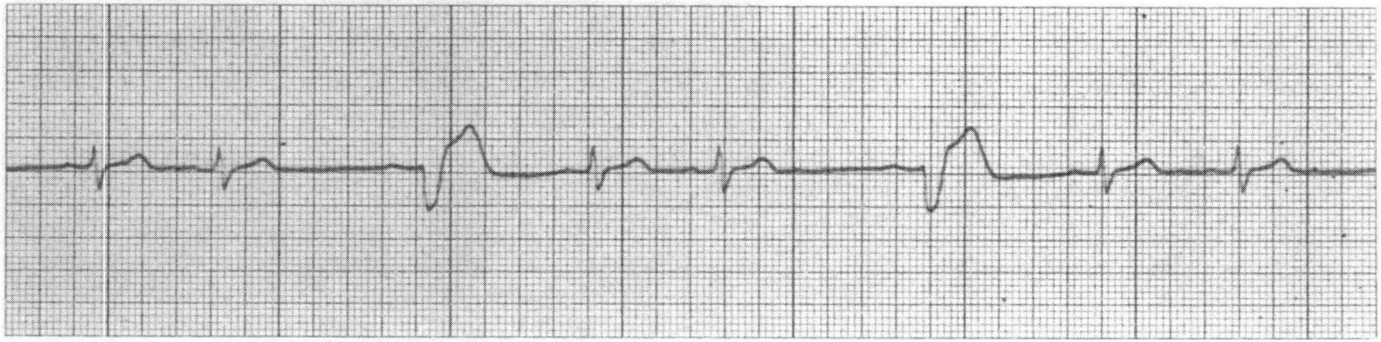

Figure 31. Bradycardia-dependent left bundle branch block (LBBB). This is much less common than rate-dependent or tachycardia-dependent LBBB. Note the P wave preceding the abnormal QRS deflection.

Torsade de Pointes (Fig. 32)

Patients with long Q–T intervals, either congenital or acquired, may develop this form of rapid, polymorphic ventricular tachycardia. Morphologically this arrhythmia is characterized by a twisting pattern of the QRS complexes, which oscillate in amplitude. The rate is usually quite rapid, and this rhythm often results in loss of consciousness or cardiac arrest. Congenital long Q–T syndrome may be associated with congenital deafness (Jervell–Lange–Nielsen syndrome) or not (Romano–Ward syndrome). Acquired long Q–T syndrome often results from electrolyte abnormalities or the use of drugs, particularly antiarrhythmic agents, that prolong the Q–T interval. (See Fig. 32.)

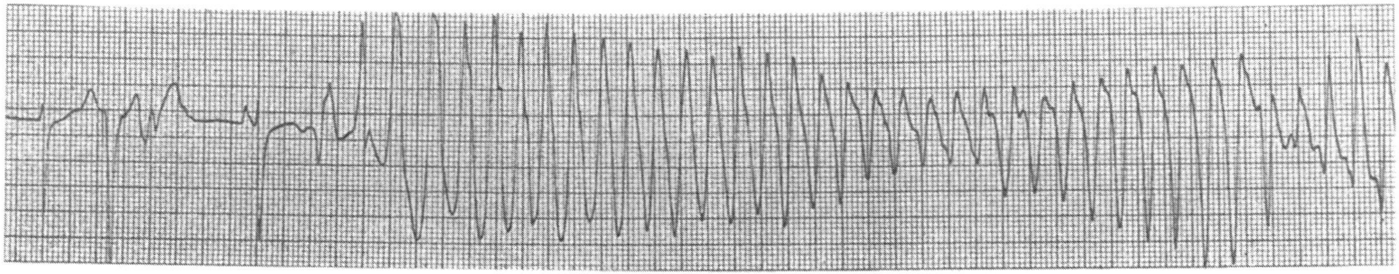

Figure 32. This single-lead tracing shows *torsade de pointes*. In the first beat of the strip the Q–T interval is 0.48 sec or greater. The QTc cannot be calculated in this tracing as it is impossible to determine the R–R interval.

Ventricular Fibrillation (Fig. 33)

Ventricular fibrillation is the most serious of the rhythm disorders, since during ventricular fibrillation no cardiac output is generated, resulting in loss of consciousness and death if defibrillation is not performed promptly. The ECG shows a fine pattern of irregular oscillations in all leads, without any discernible organized electrical activity. Figure 33 shows ventricular fibrillation. However, the fibrillatory pattern may be very fine, especially if fibrillation has been present for a long time. In that case, the tracing can look almost like a "straight line" tracing.

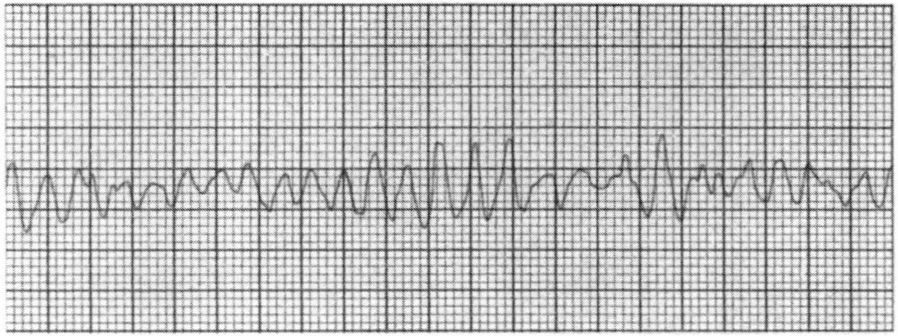

Figure 33. Ventricular fibrillation.

Irregular Ventricular Paced Rhythms (Fig. 34)

As noted earlier, some pacemakers are capable of pacing the ventricles in an irregular fashion. Usually this is the result of the pacemaker responding normally to a physiological stimulus, such as the sensed atrial rate or some other parameter designed to drive the ventricular rate according to the body's metabolic demands. Proper diagnosis requires knowing the characteristics of that patient's particular pacemaker and its normal behavior.

In many cases, pacemaker patients show a mixture of normally conducted beats and paced beats, giving rise to an irregular rhythm with at least two different QRS morphologies. This is usually evident by the presence of pacemaker spikes before the paced beats. Figure 34 shows a mixture of paced and nonpaced beats.

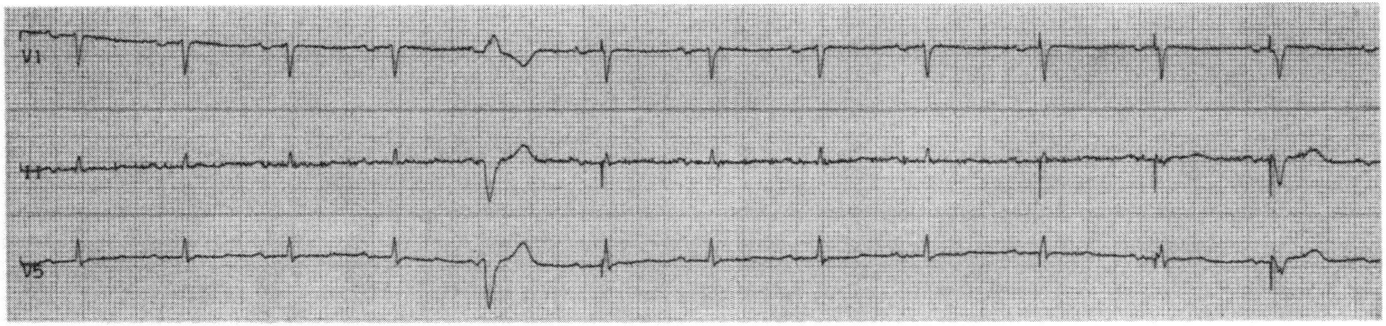

Figure 34. Three-lead rhythm strip with the final beat a paced beat. The two beats prior to the last one of the tracing are pacemaker fusion beats. The fifth complex is a PVC.

CAPTURE AS A CAUSE OF VENTRICULAR IRREGULARITY (Figs. 35 and 36)

During a regular ventricular or junctional rhythm the tracing may show occasional irregularity as a result of capture, which is the occurrence of AV conduction of atrial beats that have fallen at just the right time to conduct to the ventricle. In the case of a junctional rhythm, there will be an early, but usually unchanged, ventricular complex preceded by a P

MONITOR

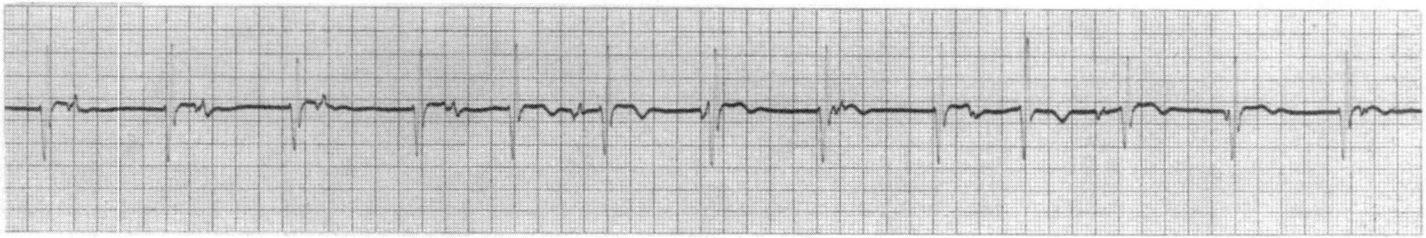

Figure 35. Accelerated junctional rhythm with isorhythmic atrioventricular (AV) dissociation. Capture of the ventricles (and AV junction) by the atrial rhythm occurs in the fifth, sixth, tenth, and eleventh complexes. The P–R intervals of the fifth and tenth beats are quite prolonged, probably owing to partial refractoriness of the AV junction following the concealed retrograde conduction from the preceding QRS complex.

wave. In the case of ventricular tachycardia, the capture will most often be seen as a narrow QRS complex which occurs when the ventricle is depolarized over the usual conducting system. Figure 35 shows a junctional rhythm with irregularity due to capture, and Figure 36 shows a ventricular tachycardia with capture.

A summary of the differential diagnosis of ventricular rhythms is given in Table 1.

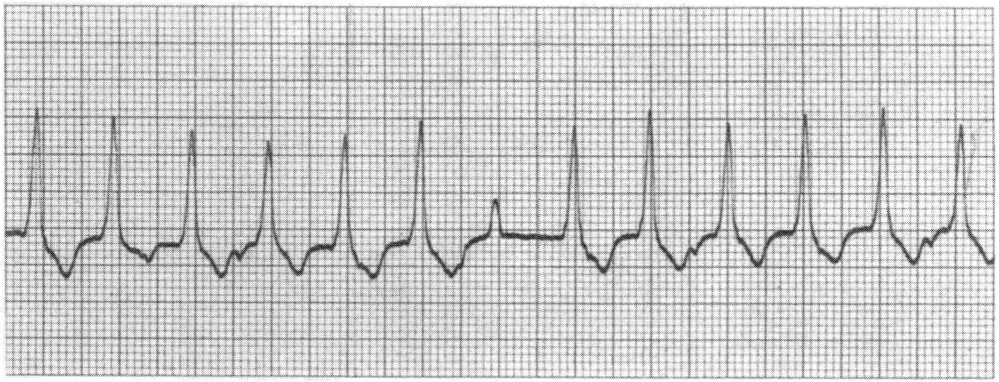

Figure 36. In this tracing the underlying rhythm is ventricular tachycardia, as indicated by atrioventricular dissociation. Capture of the 7th beat by the atrial contraction falling in the upslope of the 6th T wave is seen.

Table 1. The Differential Diagnosis of Rhythms

1. Narrow QRS complex, regular rhythm
   - A. Sinus (normal, bradycardia, or tachycardia)
   - B. Junctional (escape, accelerated, or tachycardia)
   - C. Atrial flutter, constant block
   - D. Regular atrial tachycardia due to intraatrial reentry, sinus node reentry, or automatic atrial tachycardia
   - E. Supraventricular tachycardia due to AV nodal reentry
   - F. Supraventricular tachycardia in the WPW syndrome due to orthodromic reentry (i.e., antegrade conduction over the normal conducting system with retrograde conduction over the accessory pathway)
   - E. WPW syndrome with sinus rhythm and fusion of impulses over the normal and accessory pathways
   - F. WPW syndrome with antidromic SVT (i.e., antegrade conduction over the accessory pathway, retrograde conduction over the normal pathway)
   - G. Any supraventricular rhythm with a wide QRS complex due to aberration, bundle branch block, electrolyte abnormalities, drugs, etc.
   - H. Technical problems, e.g., wrong paper speed
2. Narrow QRS complex, irregular rhythm
   - A. Sinus arrhythmia
   - B. Premature atrial complexes
   - C. Wandering atrial pacemaker
   - D. Multifocal atrial tachycardia
   - E. Sinus pauses, sinus arrest
   - F. Junctional complexes with retrograde conduction
   - G. Atrial flutter with variable block
   - H. Atrial fibrillation
3. Wide QRS complex, regular rhythm
   - A. Ventricular escape rhythm
   - B. Accelerated idioventricular rhythm
   - C. Ventricular tachycardia
   - D. Ventricular paced rhythms
4. Wide QRS, irregular rhythm
   - A. Premature ventricular complexes
   - B. *Torsade de pointes*
   - C. Ventricular fibrillation
   - D. Irregular ventricular paced rhythms or rhythms that are a mixture of paced and unpaced beats
   - E. Capture beats interrupting a regular ventricular or junctional rhythm
   - F. Atrial fibrillation that is conducted to the ventricles over an accessory pathway in a patient with WPW syndrome
   - G. Any irregular supraventricular arrhythmia associated with a wide QRS complex due to aberration, bundle branch block, electrolyte abnormalities, or drug effects
5. No organized ventricular activity
   - A. Fine ventricular fibrillation
   - B. Asystole
   - C. Technical errors

DISTINGUISHING VENTRICULAR FROM SUPRAVENTRICULAR ARRHYTHMIAS (Fig. 37)

One of the most challenging tasks in electrocardiography is determining whether a sustained tachycardia is supraventricular, and generally less dangerous, or ventricular in origin, with a higher risk.

The best way to determine whether a tachycardia is ventricular or supraventricular is to begin by asking two questions:

1. Are the QRS complexes of normal or near-normal morphology?
2. What is the relationship between the P waves and the QRS complexes?

If the QRS complexes are narrow (<0.12 sec), and particularly if they are identical to the QRS complexes during normal sinus rhythm, then the arrhythmia is most likely supraventricular. If the QRS complexes are wide, the rhythm is likely to be ventricular in origin. These principles, unfortunately, are not always true. Some ventricular tachycardias may have a narrow QRS complex, and occasionally the QRS of ventricular tachycardia mimics the QRS seen during sinus rhythm. Conversely, supraventricular tachycardias may be conducted to the ventricles with aberrancy and result in a wide-QRS-complex tachycardia. The possibility of this occurrence has been overemphasized, since the most common cause of sustained wide-QRS-complex tachycardia is ventricular tachycardia. Wide-QRS-complex tachycardias should be considered to be ventricular tachycardia unless there is good evidence to the contrary.

The relationship between P waves and QRS complexes in this setting can be either very helpful or not helpful at all. Unfortunately, it is frequently difficult to see P waves.

If, during a wide-QRS-complex tachycardia, there is clear-cut AV dissociation, with P waves seen independent of and at a different rate than the QRS complexes, then the rhythm is *not* supraventricular and must arise from the ventricles. This is very helpful diagnostically.

If there is a P wave associated with each QRS

complex, then the arrhythmia may be *either* ventricular tachycardia with retrograde conduction of each beat back to the atria, *or* supraventricular tachycardia with antegrade conduction of each supraventricular beat to the ventricles. The finding of a 1:1 AV relationship is thus not very helpful diagnostically.

The setting in which the rhythm occurs is sometimes helpful. When abnormal beats or a wide-QRS-complex tachycardia occurs in a patient with organic heart disease, particularly in the patient with previous myocardial infarction, a ventricular origin of the arrhythmia is much more likely.

One absolute criterion for stating that a rhythm is ventricular in origin is the presence of ventricular fusion beats. This phenomenon occurs when the P waves are dissociated from the tachycardia itself, and a P wave fortuitously falls at a time when it is able to conduct antegrade over the normal conducting system. The result will be fusion of a supraventricular beat with a beat of ventricular origin. This will result in a narrower QRS complex than beats of ventricular origin and a configuration of the QRS that is intermediate between that resulting from a supraventricular beat and that resulting from an ventricular focus.

Figures 22 and 37 both show ventricular rhythms with fusion beats. The merging of the two ECG patterns resulting from the nearly simultaneous discharge of two pacemakers is clearly evident. A similar phenomenon is seen in Figure 34, where pacemaker fusion beats are seen, in this case with the underlying rhythm being supraventricular and the pacemaker impulses simulating a ventricular focus of depolarization.

The phenomenon of capture can also help in the diagnosis of a dysrhythmia. Capture is the disruption of a rhythm by a discharge from another, higher, focus. The presence of capture can be useful in demonstrating that a series of complexes is of either supraventricular or ventricular origin. For example, if a rhythm is reset forward by a fortuitously placed P wave that is conducted, then "capture" of the rhythm by an atrial discharge has occurred. If there is no change in the waveform of the complexes when capture occurs, then the basic rhythm must have a supraventricular origin. If, however, the "captured" beat has a different waveform, then the underlying rhythm is more likely ventricular in origin. Figure 35 shows capture of a junctional rhythm and Figure 36 shows capture of a ventricular tachycardia.

Table 2 gives some general guidelines for determining the origin of wide-QRS-complex tachycardias.[12,13]

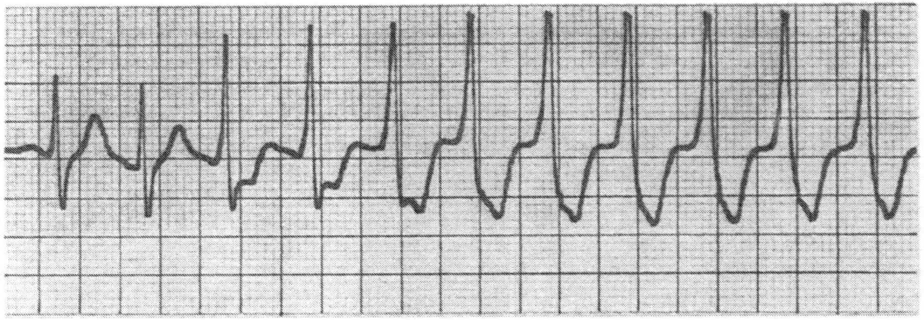

Figure 37. A run of ventricular tachycardia. The 3rd, 4th, and 5th complexes show progressive fusion between the sinus rhythm morphology and the ventricular tachycardia.

Table 2. Wide QRS Complex Tachycardias: Distinguishing Ventricular from Supraventricular Tachycardia

1. *AV dissociation:* Dissociated atrial activity is strongly suggestive of ventricular tachycardia.
2. *Fusion beats:* The presence of fusion beats proves two separate foci and, if present, the wide QRS beats must be ventricular in origin unless an artificial pacemaker is present.
3. *Capture:* The occurrence of capture by the atria suggests supraventricular origin of a dysrhythmia *if* the waveform of the QRS is unchanged when capture occurs. If capture occurs and the captured QRS complex is narrow, the wide-complex tachycardia is probably ventricular.
4. *Wide QRS:* A QRS complex of greater than 0.14 sec (or greater than 0.14 sec for RBBB morphology tachycardias and greater than 0.16 sec for LBBB morphology tachycardias) suggests ventricular tachycardia.
5. *Concordance of QRS:* Concordance of QRS complexes in the precordial leads (all QRS complexes largely positive or negative) suggests ventricular tachycardia.
6. *Left axis:* Left-axis deviation is uncommon in supraventricular tachycardias and suggests ventricular tachycardia.
7. *Irregularly irregular rhythm:* A wide-complex tachycardia that is irregularly irregular suggests atrial fibrillation or multifocal atrial tachycardia, either conducted over an accessory pathway or conducted with ventricular aberration. Atrial flutter with variable block and aberrant conduction could also give a grossly irregular wide-complex ventricular rhythm.
8. *Known or suspected heart disease:* A wide-complex tachycardia, occurring in the setting of known structural heart disease, particularly previous myocardial infarction, suggests ventricular tachycardia.

VENTRICULAR RHYTHMS AND ATRIOVENTRICULAR BLOCK

Introduction

Forms of atrioventricular block that affect the cardiac rhythm are second-degree AV block (either Mobitz I or Mobitz II) and third-degree AV block. First-degree AV block, which is simply prolongation of the P–R interval, is discussed later under abnormalities of the P–R interval.

Second- and third-degree AV block may be diagnosed when a P wave that would otherwise be expected to conduct fails to conduct to the ventricles. Thus, the failure of a premature atrial complex that falls soon after the preceding QRS to conduct to the ventricles does not necessarily mean that AV block is present, since the AV junction may have been still refractory from the preceding discharge.

However, a normally timed P wave that fails to conduct is evidence of AV block. In first-degree AV block, all the normally timed P waves conduct to the ventricles, but with a long P–R interval. In second-degree AV block, some P waves conduct and some do not. Second-degree block can be further subdivided into Mobitz type I and Mobitz type II block. In third-degree AV block, none of the P waves are conducted.

Mobitz Type I (Wenckebach) Second-Degree AV Block (Figs. 38 and 39)

Mobitz type I (Wenckebach) block is characterized by P–R intervals that increase with each succeeding cycle until finally there is nonconduction of one of the P waves. Because the lengthening of each P–R interval is less than the amount by which the preceding interval was lengthened, there is a decrease in the R–R intervals with each cycle until one is dropped and the process starts over. The presence of grouped beating—clusters of QRS complexes separated by pauses—should alert the reader to the possibility of Mobitz type I block. Mobitz type I block is more common in inferior myocardial infarctions and in patients with drug effects. Occasionally, normal people with a high level of vagal tone exhibit Mobitz type I second-degree AV block. Mobitz type I block most often occurs at the level of the AV node. Figures 38 and 39 show Mobitz I block.

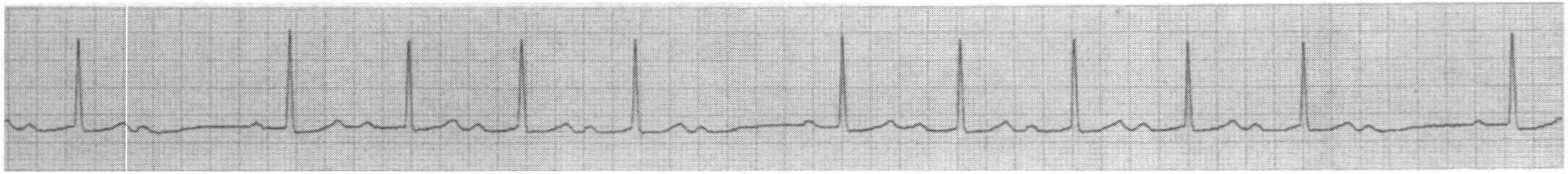

Figure 38. Monitor tracing of Mobitz type I atrioventricular block (Wenckebach). The P–R intervals progressively lengthen and the R–R intervals shorten in the classic manner.

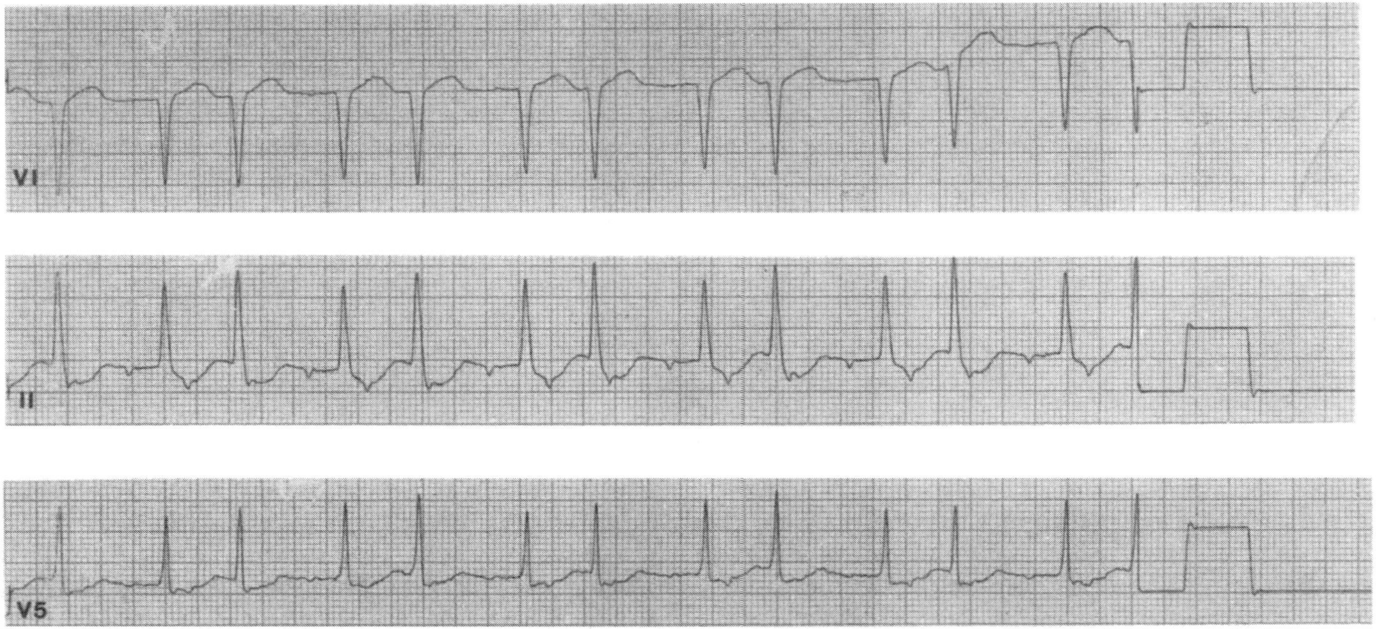

Figure 39. Three-lead monitor tracing of Mobitz type I atrioventricular (AV) block. The rhythm is an ectopic atrial tachycardia with a rate of about 170. A 3:2 AV block is present. It is possible to demonstrate that this is Mobitz I block as the P–R intervals are consistently shorter after the dropped P wave than before.

Mobitz Type II Second-Degree AV Block (Figs. 40 and 41)

In Mobitz type II block, the failure of conduction is abrupt and without warning, with no previous prolongation of the P–R interval. This is a more serious form of AV block, as it is a common forerunner of third-degree AV block and tends to occur in more seriously ill patients. If there is fixed 2:1 AV block, it is not possible to differentiate between Mobitz type I block and Mobitz type II, since there are never two consecutive P–R intervals for comparison. Mobitz type II block is more common in the setting of anterior myocardial infarction and in the presence of preexisting bundle branch block. Most frequently, the site of block is in the His–Purkinje system. Figures 40 and 41 show Mobitz type II block.

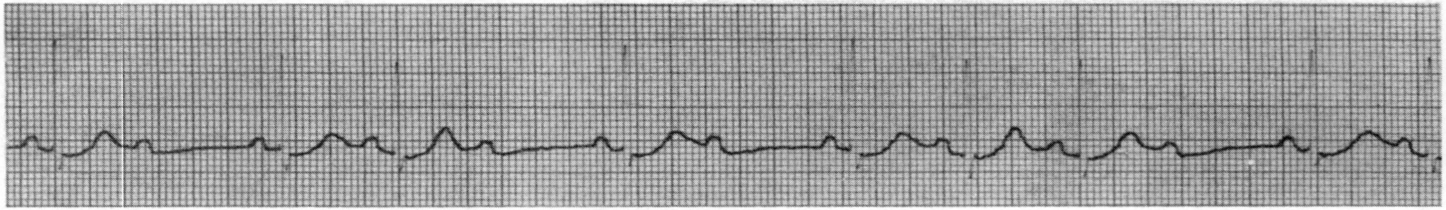

Figure 40. Monitor tracing showing Mobitz type II atrioventricular block. The second, fifth, seventh, and eleventh P waves do not conduct, yet the P–R interval is otherwise unchanged throughout the tracing.

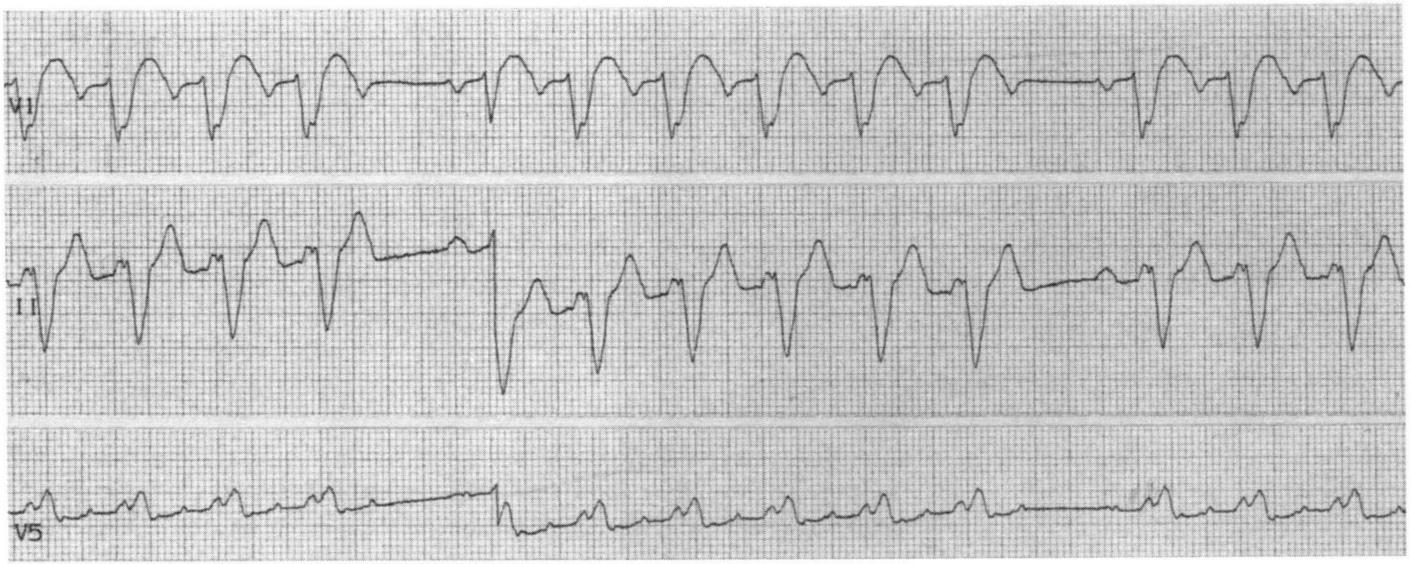

Figure 41. Three-lead rhythm strip showing Mobitz type II atrioventricular (AV) block. This is a more difficult strip to read as most of the P waves are obscured by the preceding T waves. However, in V5, small P waves can be clearly seen and the diagnosis of Mobitz type II AV block can be made as the P–R intervals do not change after the dropped P wave.

Third-Degree AV Block (Fig. 42)

Third-degree AV block is present when there is complete failure of atrial activity to conduct to the ventricles at a time when normal conduction would be expected to occur. When the expected conduction does not occur, there may be AV dissociation *due to* third-degree AV block. Figure 42 shows AV dissociation due to third-degree AV block. In this tracing AV block is proved by the absence of AV conduction even when P waves occur at times when conduction would be expected.

However, AV dissociation can occur in the absence of third-degree AV block. For example, if the rate of an accelerated pacemaker in the junction or ventricle exceeds the atrial rate, dissociation without AV block can occur. This is shown in Figures 11, 35, and 36. In Figure 36 it can be shown that even though AV dissociation is present, third-degree AV block is not, since one atrial beat does conduct in the expected manner.

When AV dissociation is present, it is common for there to be an apparent relationship between atrial and ventricular activity. This can happen even in the presence of third-degree AV block if the atria and ventricles are beating in coincidental synchrony. This is called isorhythmic AV dissociation. Figure 35 shows isorhythmic AV dissociation.

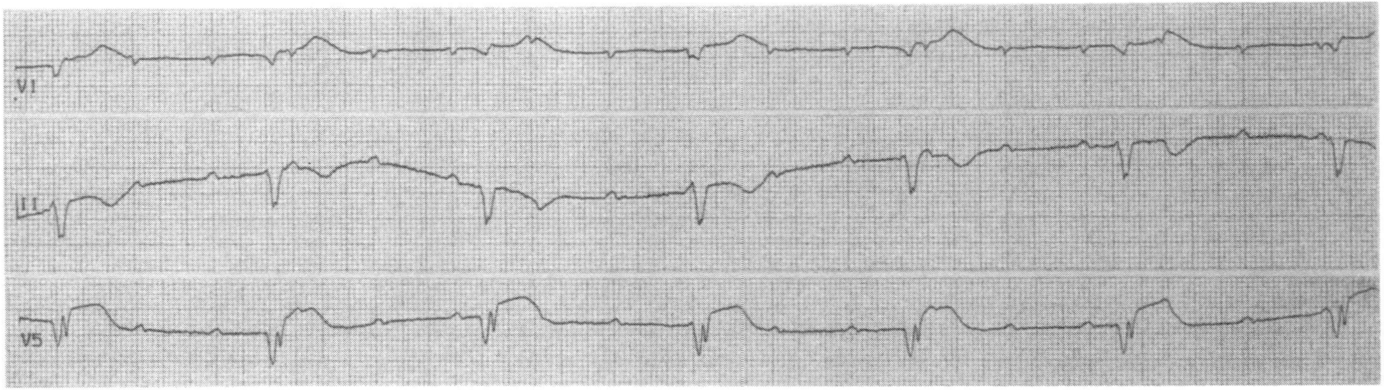

Figure 42. Three-lead rhythm strip showing atrioventricular (AV) dissociation due to third-degree AV block. There is atrial activity with a rate of 100 and a ventricular escape rhythm with a rate of 37. There is no relationship between the two.

6

Abnormalities of Conduction (Exclusive of Second- and Third-Degree Atrioventricular Block)

In cases where the intervals are all prolonged, especially if an apparent bradycardia is present, it is necessary to find out whether the paper speed was set correctly, since recording the electrocardiogram (ECG) at a 50 mm/sec paper speed instead of the usual 25 mm/sec will cause apparent lengthening of the intervals. Abnormalities of conduction manifesting as alterations in the cardiac rhythm were discussed in Chapter 5. Alterations in the axis, which can also be caused by abnormalities of conduction, are discussed in this chapter.

ABNORMALITIES OF THE P–R INTERVAL

Introduction

The P–R interval is measured between the beginning of the P wave and the onset of the QRS complex and in many cases is actually a "P–Q" interval. In adults the normal P–R interval is between 0.12 and 0.20 sec, with some variability due to rate. At slow heart rates (below 70) a P–R interval of 0.21 sec would not suggest AV block, while at rapid heart rates a "normal" P–R interval of 0.20 sec might be abnormal. In adults, it can be assumed that a P–R interval of 0.10 sec or less suggests that the atrial beat did not conduct normally to the ventricles. The explanation would then be that there was an accessory pathway, as in WPW syndrome, an abnormally rapid AV conduction time, as in Lown–Ganong–Levine syndrome, or retrograde conduction from a junctional beat, or that the timing was a coincidence of two unrelated events such as a sinus beat and a premature junctional beat.

First-Degree Atrioventricular Block (Fig. 43)

P–R intervals greater than 0.20 or 0.21 sec represent first-degree atrioventricular (AV) block. This prolongation of the P–R interval may be due to a variety of factors:

1. Bradycardia (modest prolongation of the P–R interval is normal with bradycardia)
2. Enhanced vagal tone

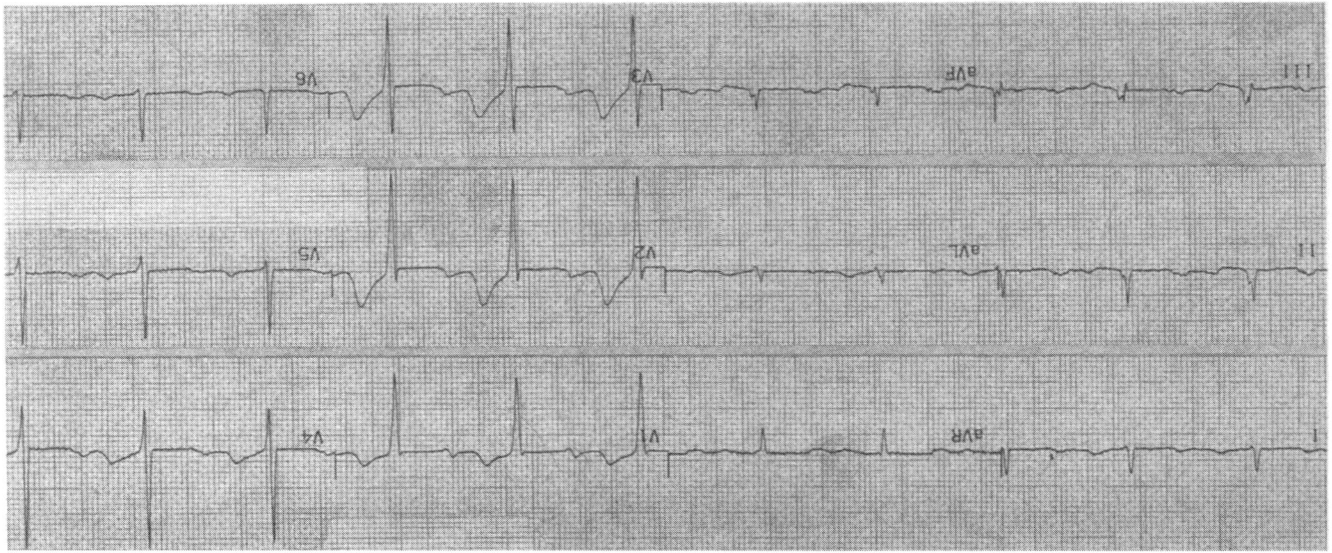

Figure 43. Marked first-degree atrioventricular block with a P–R interval of 0.42 sec. Other than minor T-wave abnormalities the tracing is normal. Note that in the lateral leads the P waves simulate U waves.

3. Drugs (e.g., digitalis, calcium channel blockers, beta blockers)
4. Hyperkalemia
5. Pathological changes in the conducting system (e.g., fibrosis, ischemia, infarction, or inflammation as in rheumatic fever)

Figures 43 and 44 show first-degree AV block. Note that in Figure 43, although the P–R interval is quite long (0.42 sec), the consistent relationship between the P waves and the QRS complexes suggests that AV conduction is indeed taking place.

Variable P–R intervals occur with atrial contractions arising from differing foci, as is the case with PACs or multifocal atrial tachycardia, or may be seen as part of the Wenckebach phenomenon. Figures 15 and 16 show variable P–R intervals resulting from wandering atrial pacemaker and a multifocal atrial rhythm.

ABNORMALITIES OF THE QRS INTERVAL (INCLUDING BUNDLE BRANCH BLOCKS)

Introduction

The normal QRS interval in adults is between 0.08 and 0.10 sec measured from the first inflection of the initial Q or R wave to the J point which marks the termination of the QRS complex and the start of the ST segment. The QRS complex may be prolonged by the presence of right or left bundle branch block (RBBB, LBBB), nonspecific delays in intraventricular conduction, electrolyte abnormalities, or drug effects. Chapter 5 gives the differential diagnosis of rhythms with prolonged QRS complexes and the same differential diagnosis is relevant here. The fascicular blocks are discussed in Chapter 9.

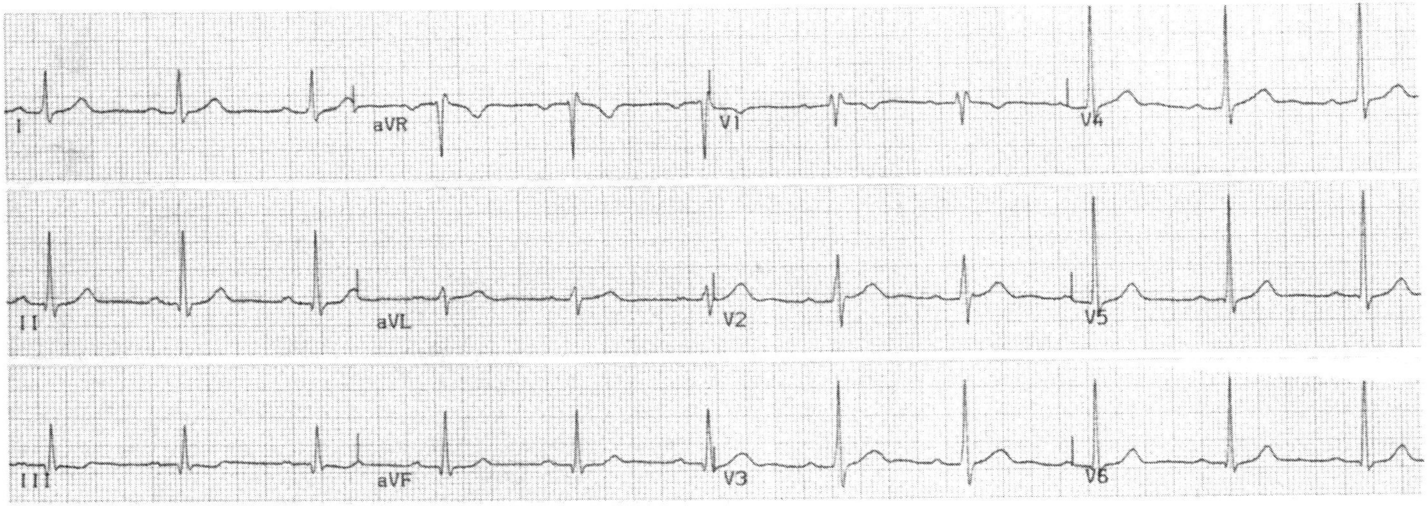

Figure 44. Incomplete right bundle branch block with QRS of 0.10 to 0.11 sec and first-degree atrioventricular block with P–R interval of 0.21 sec.

Right Bundle Branch Block (Figs. 44 and 45)

In RBBB the depolarization of the right ventricle is delayed, but septal depolarization and depolarization of the left ventricle are not delayed. Thus, the effects of RBBB are seen mainly in the visualization of right ventricular forces which were previously obscured by the left ventricular depolarization. The right ventricular forces are now seen late in the cardiac cycle. Thus, terminal positive forces are seen in V1 and sometimes in V2 (the classic rSR′ pattern, which is the hallmark of RBBB), and in aVR. A slurred S wave seen in leads I, aVL, and V6 represents the delayed right ventricular depolarization vector moving away from the superior and lateral leads. The ST segments and T waves (which arise primarily from the normally depolarizing left ventricle) are not markedly changed and those changes which are present are confined mainly to the right precordium. Complete RBBB has a QRS duration of 0.12 sec or greater, and if incomplete the duration is between 0.10 and 0.12 sec. Figure 44 shows incomplete RBBB and Figure 45 shows complete RBBB. The QRS duration is 0.11 sec in the first tracing and 0.14 sec in the second tracing.

An rSR′ pattern in V1 may also be seen in other conditions. The differential diagnosis of the rSR′ in V1 should include the following conditions:

1. Normal variant (if QRS is 0.10 sec or less)
2. Incomplete or complete RBBB
3. Posterior myocardial infarction
4. Right ventricular hypertrophy
5. Chronic obstructive pulmonary disease and/or cor pulmonale

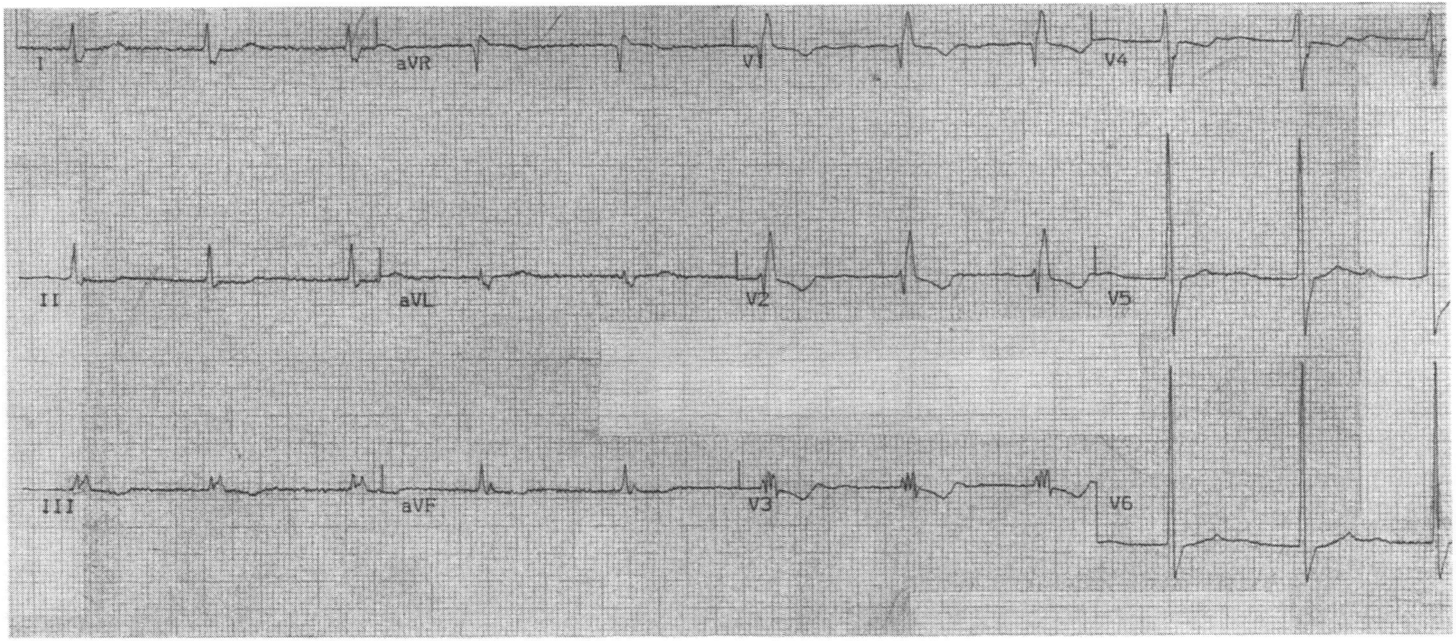

Figure 45. Complete right bundle branch block with a QRS of 0.12 sec. The rhythm is atrial fibrillation. The ventricular response is slightly irregular.

Left Bundle Branch Block (Figs. 46 and 47)

The LBBB pattern is more bizarre than the RBBB pattern since the major mass of the ventricles is involved in the abnormal conduction. Changes due to LBBB are more widespread and prominently include the ST segment and the T wave. In patients without bundle branch block, normal septal depolarization occurs from left to right since the left side of the septum is activated first by the left bundle branch, resulting in normal "septal Q waves" in the lateral leads. In LBBB septal depolarization occurs from right to left and these septal Q waves are lost. Normal right ventricular forces are nearly lost in the abnormal depolarization of the left ventricle, seen mainly as initial R waves in the right precordial leads. Deep rS or QS complexes become broad and slurred R wave complexes as one moves from the right to the left precordial leads. Similarly, the limb leads show broad and slurred complexes and the ST segments merge with the wide and inverted T waves. In complete LBBB the QRS duration is 0.12 sec or more. If the block is incomplete, the QRS duration is between 0.10 and 0.12 sec. Figures 46 and 47 show complete LBBB. LBBB can occur with or without left-axis deviation, as shown in these two figures. In addition, Figure 19 shows LBBB with left-axis deviation of about $-60°$.

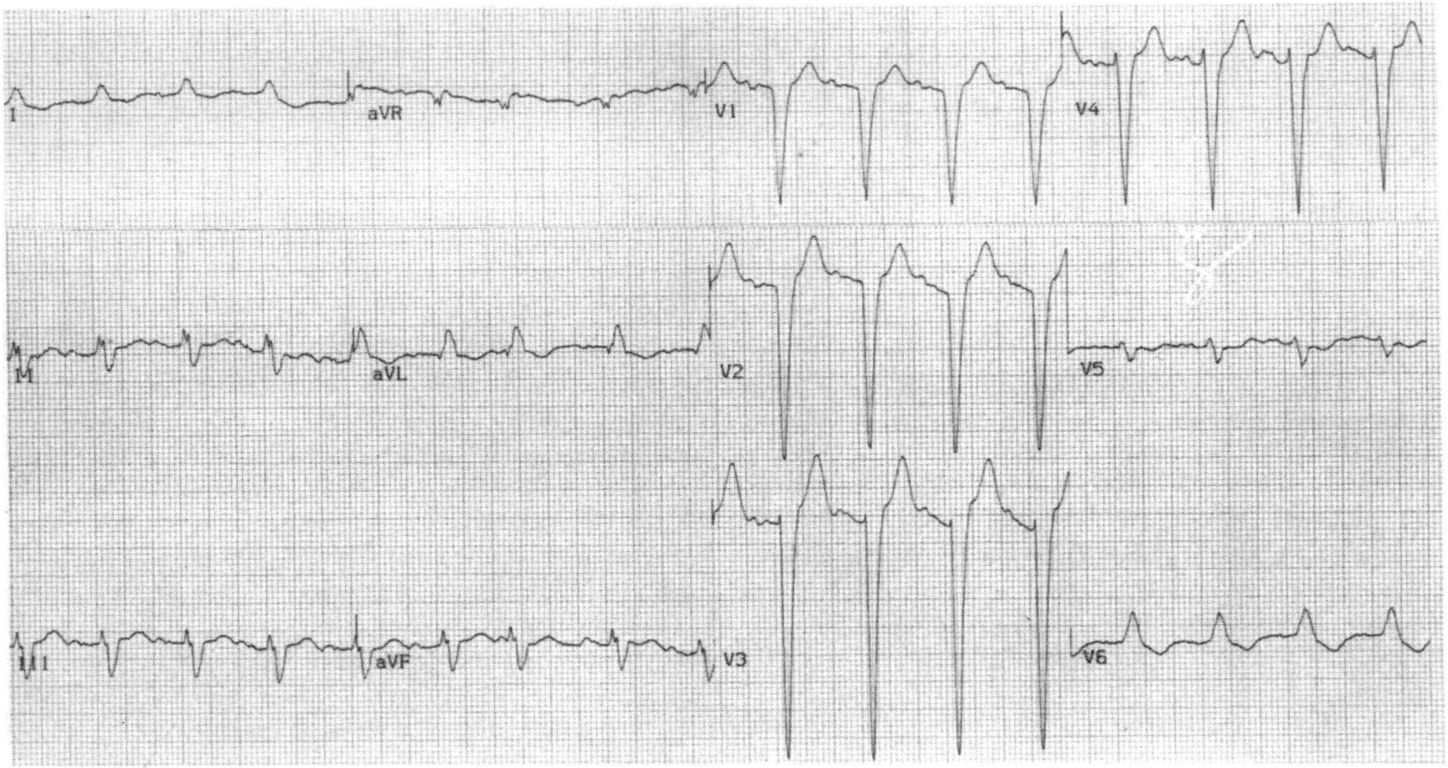

Figure 46. Complete left bundle branch block. One PAC occurs as the 7th complex. The axis is −30°.

Abnormalities of the Ventricular Intrinsicoid Deflection

The intrinsicoid deflection, also called the ventricular activation time, is the time measured from the onset of the Q wave to the peak of the R wave (or the onset of the R wave to the peak of the R wave if no Q is present) in a precordial lead with a dominant R wave. The intrinsicoid deflection time should be less than 0.05 sec in lateral precordial leads in the normal adult. Increases in the time to the intrinsicoid deflection time are related to abnormal conduction patterns, such as bundle branch block, myocardial infarction, or ventricular hypertrophy, which increase the length of time required for ventricular depolarization. Figure 47 shows a prolonged intrinsicoid deflection time due to LBBB.

Nonspecific Intraventricular Conduction Delay

Patients may have wide QRS complexes during normal rhythm and yet not have the criteria for either complete right or left bundle branch block. This phenomenon is most often seen in patients with cardiomyopathy or extensive coronary disease with previous infarction and may also be seen as a result of electrolyte disturbances or drug effects. In this case the electrocardiogram is usually read as a nonspecific intraventricular conduction delay.

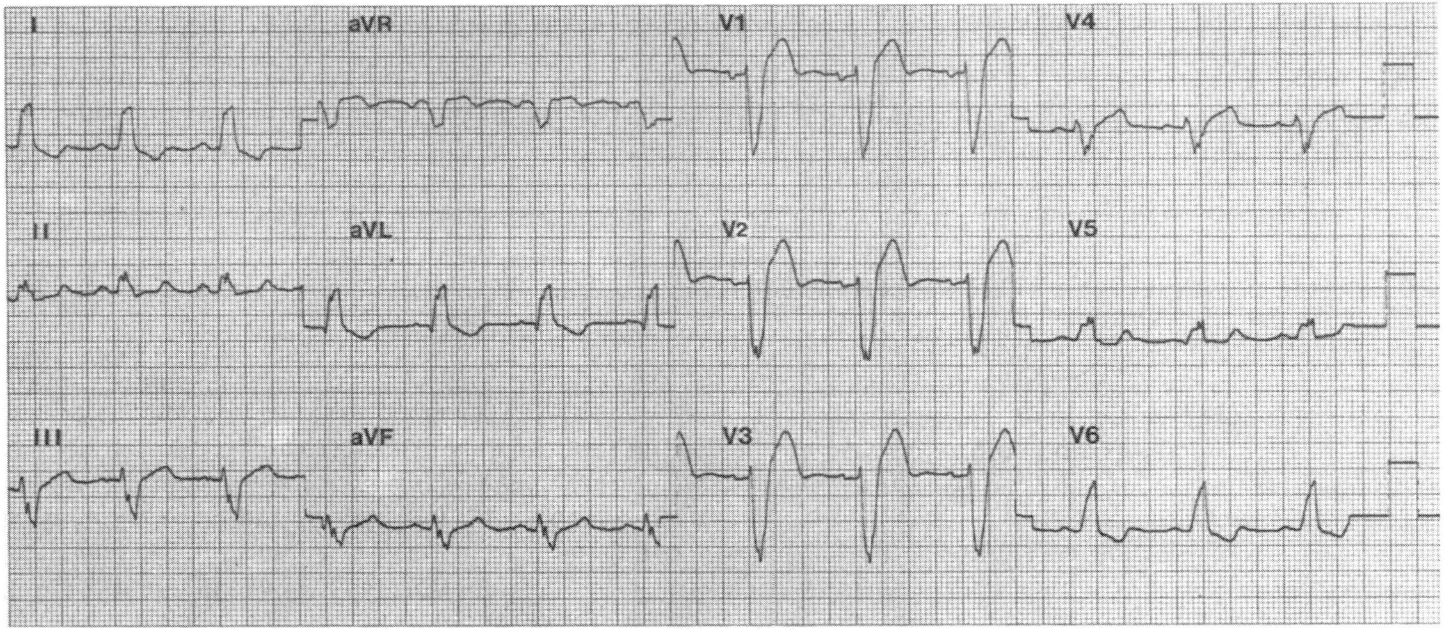

Figure 47. Complete left bundle branch block. The axis is 0°.

ABNORMALITIES OF THE Q–T INTERVAL

The Q–T interval is measured from the beginning of the QRS complex until the termination of the T wave. Before it can be decided that the Q–T interval is normal or abnormal, it is necessary to calculate the corrected Q–T interval or Q–Tc if the rate is far from 60. The normal Q–T interval is between 0.35 and 0.44 sec, depending on heart rate, and the upper limit of the Q–Tc is 0.42 to 0.43 sec. The Q–Tc is calculated by dividing the Q–T interval in seconds by the square root of the R–R interval in seconds.

$$\text{Q–Tc} = \frac{\text{Q–T (seconds)}}{\sqrt{\text{R–R (seconds)}}}$$

Thus, when the rate = 60, the Q–T is equal to the Q–Tc since that rate corresponds to an R–R interval of 1 sec.

The differential diagnosis of the abnormally short Q–T interval includes the following:

1. Thyrotoxicosis
2. Hypercalcemia
3. Digitalis toxicity

In the case of hypercalcemia, the shortening of the Q–T interval is really due to a shortening of the ST segment, thus giving rise to a T wave that arises directly from the end of the QRS complex.

The differential diagnosis of the abnormally long Q–T interval includes the following:

1. Drugs (especially type IA antiarrhythmic drugs such as quinidine)
2. Electrolyte disturbances (hypocalcemia, hypomagnesemia)
3. Conduction defects (bundle branch blocks, intraventricular conduction defects)
4. Myocardial disease (infarction, hypertrophy, myocarditis)
5. Cerebral disease (especially acute intracerebral hemorrhage)
6. Hypothermia
7. Hereditary long Q–T syndromes, including Jervell–Lange–Nielsen and Romano–Ward syndromes.
8. Paper speed set incorrectly
9. Hypokalemia (apparent rather than real prolongation)

Hypokalemia probably results in a prolonged Q–T interval because of flattening of the T wave and the presence of a more prominent U wave, and thus the Q–U interval is prolonged. Hypocalcemia causes a prolongation mainly of the S–T interval and this causes prolongation of the Q–T. A prolonged Q–T interval, either congenital or acquired, may predispose the patient to a particularly refractory form of ventricular tachycardia called *torsade de pointes*. Individuals with the hereditary form of prolonged QT syndrome have, in the absence of treatment, a 1–2% annual mortality rate from sudden death as a result of *torsade de pointes* culminating in ventricular fibrillation.[13]

7

Abnormalities of the Electrical Axis

INTRODUCTION

The axis is the direction in the frontal plane of the net vector of electrical activity, whether the P wave, QRS complex, or T wave. However, "axis" usually refers to the QRS axis. As previously noted, the axis can be measured by determining the lead in which the sum of the areas over and under the baseline is zero. The vector is thus perpendicular to this lead and must be in one of two directions. By examining the lead at right angles to this lead and noting whether the complex in question is largely positive or largely negative in that lead, one can easily determine the direction of the axis. In some cases, no realistic estimate of the axis in the frontal plane can be made, and the axis is said to be indeterminate.

ABNORMALITIES OF THE P-WAVE AXIS

In the frontal plane the P wave normally has an axis of approximately $+30°$ to $+60°$ and the vector points slightly anteriorly. The usual P wave is therefore upright in limb lead II, and deviation from this rule is expected only in the event of

1. Lead misplacement (right and left arms reversed)
2. Ectopic atrial focus or junctional rhythm
3. Dextrocardia

Right- and left-axis deviation of the P wave can occur in right and left atrial abnormalities or enlargement, in a variety of other conditions, and in normal persons.

ABNORMALITIES OF THE QRS AXIS

The QRS axis represents the sum of the major electrical forces resulting from ventricular depolarization.

Left-Axis Deviation

Left-axis deviation is generally defined as an electrical axis in the frontal plane which is leftward (really superior) of $-30°$. The causes of left-axis deviation include the following conditions. Figure 19 shows left-axis deviation.

1. Normal variant
2. Left anterior fascicular block
3. Inferior wall myocardial infarction
4. WPW syndrome, especially with posterior septal accessory pathways
5. Myocarditis
6. Left ventricular hypertrophy (LVH)
7. Left bundle branch block (LBBB) and incomplete left bundle branch block (ILBBB)

Although LBBB, ILBBB, and LVH can be associated with left-axis deviation, they do not necessarily cause it. When LVH is present, the axis will only rarely be rightward.

Left Anterior Fascicular Block (Figs. 48 and 49)

Block that is confined to the anterior or posterior fascicles of the left bundle branch presents as deviation in the QRS axis rather than QRS prolongation. The criteria for left anterior fascicular block (also called left anterior hemiblock) include an initial vector that is directed posteriorly, inferiorly, and to the right. However, since the left anterior fascicle is an anterior and superior structure, the net direction of ventricular depolarization, which must start at the left posterior fascicle, is upward or to the left, and the net QRS axis is shifted to −30° or more. A large R wave should be present in aVL.

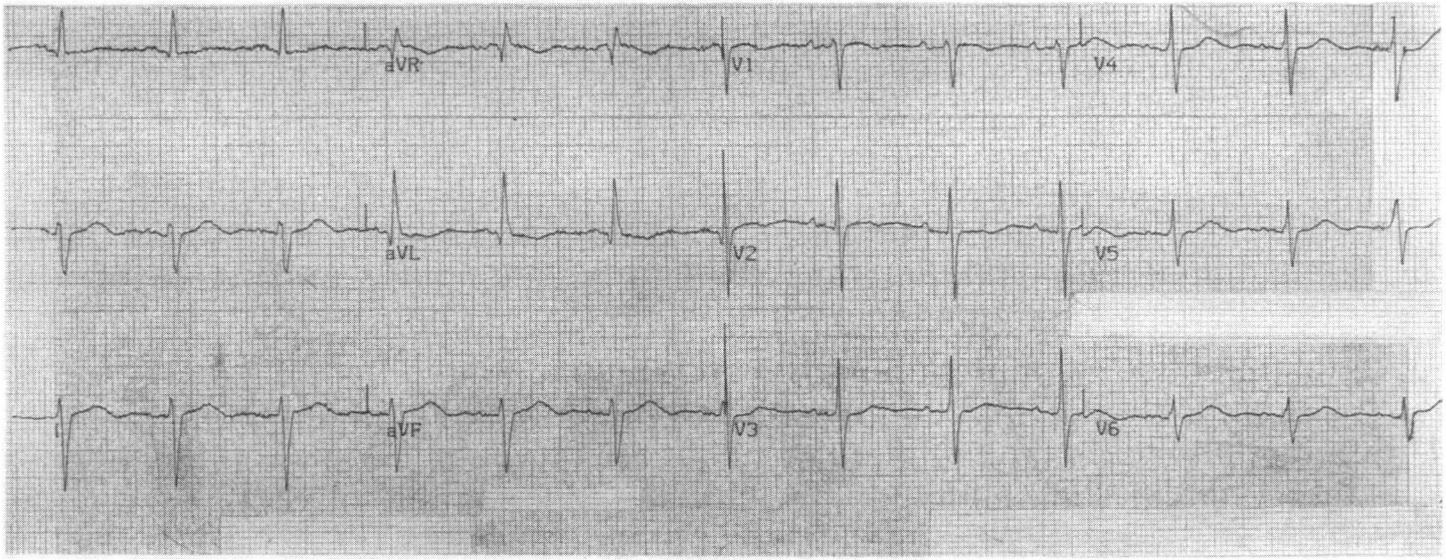

Figure 48. Left-axis deviation due to left anterior fascicular block. Note the large R waves in aVL and the small Q waves in I and aVL. The axis is −60°.

Left anterior fascicular block (LAFB) can be initially recognized by the net negative QRS complexes in the inferior leads, with an S wave being greater than the R wave in lead II. The initial vector will produce small R waves in the inferior leads (if there has been no infarction) and small Q waves in I and aVL. Unless there is QRS widening from some other cause, the QRS interval should be normal. However, it is necessary to differentiate the left-axis deviation due to LAFB from that due to other causes such as inferior wall infarction.

Figures 48 and 49 show tracings with left-axis deviation of about $-60°$ due to different causes. Figure 48 shows the effects of LAFB and Figure 49 shows left-axis deviation due to an inferior wall myocardial infarction.

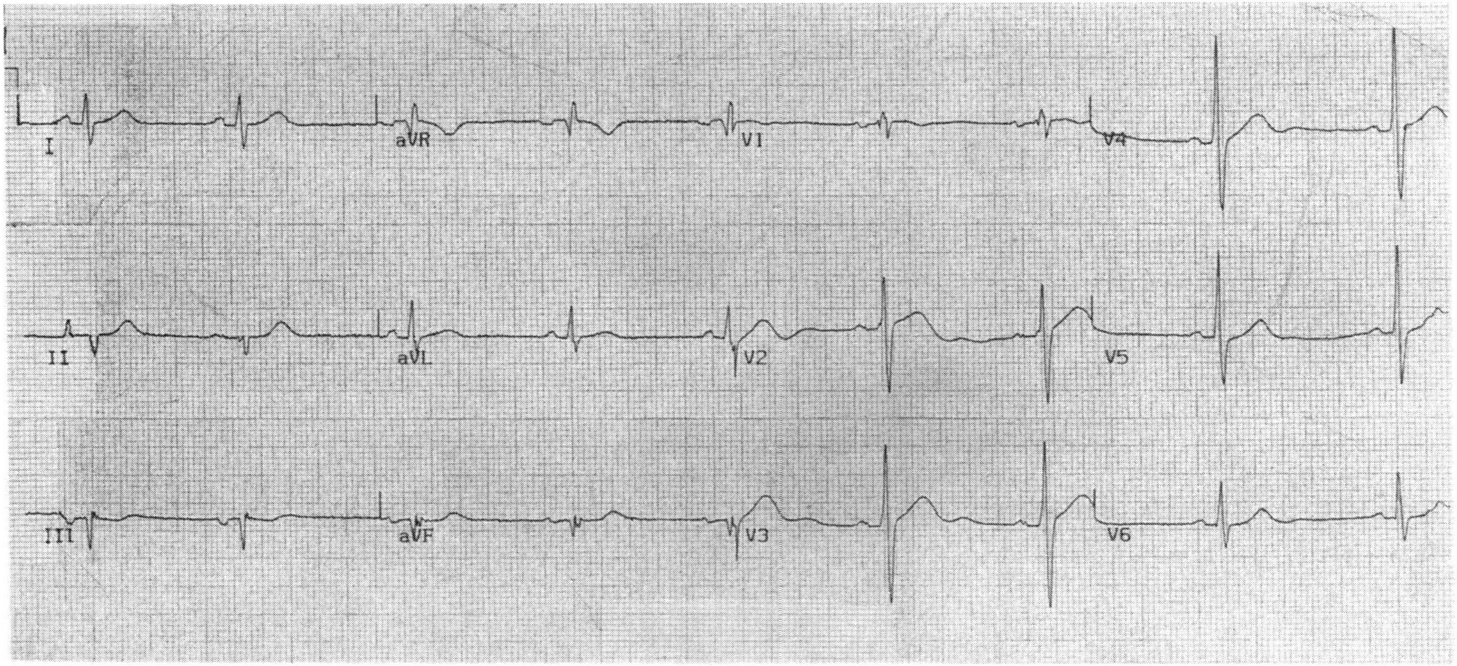

Figure 49. Left-axis deviation of $-60°$ due to inferior wall myocardial infarction. Note the Q waves in leads II, III, and aVF.

Right-Axis Deviation (Fig. 50)

Right-axis deviation exists when the frontal plane axis is greater than or equal to +110°. The causes of right-axis deviation include the following conditions:

1. Normal variant
2. Right ventricular hypertrophy
3. Left posterior fascicular block
4. Chronic obstructive pulmonary disease (COPD) and/or cor pulmonale
5. Superior wall or anterolateral wall infarction
6. Dextrocardia
7. Vertical heart
8. Lead misplacement (reversal of right and left arm leads)

Figure 50 shows right-axis deviation to about +180° due to anterosuperior infarction.

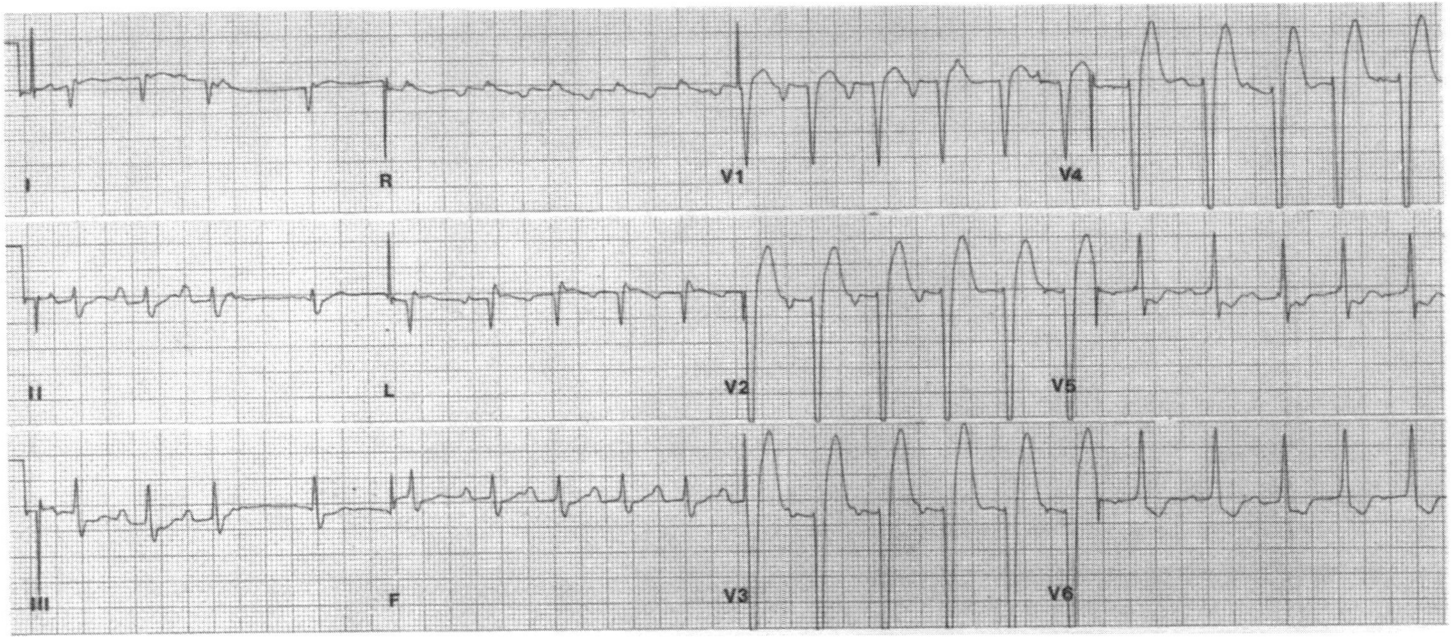

Figure 50. Right-axis deviation due to anterosuperior myocardial infarction. Q waves are seen in leads I and aVL. The axis is between +150° and +180° and there is a blocked PAC after the third QRS complex followed by a junctional escape beat.

Left Posterior Fascicular Block (Fig. 51)

This form of fascicular block, also called left posterior hemiblock, is much less common than LAFB. As would be expected, the effects on the QRS complex are roughly opposite to those found in LAFB. The axis is rightward, usually in the range of +120°. There are initial R waves in I and aVL and initial short (0.02 sec) Q waves in the inferior leads. The R wave in lead III is usually greater than the R wave in lead II, reflecting the far rightward axis. The other causes of right axis deviation listed earlier (especially lead misplacement) should be excluded before the diagnosis of left posterior fascicular block (LPFB) is made. Figure 51 shows LPFB.

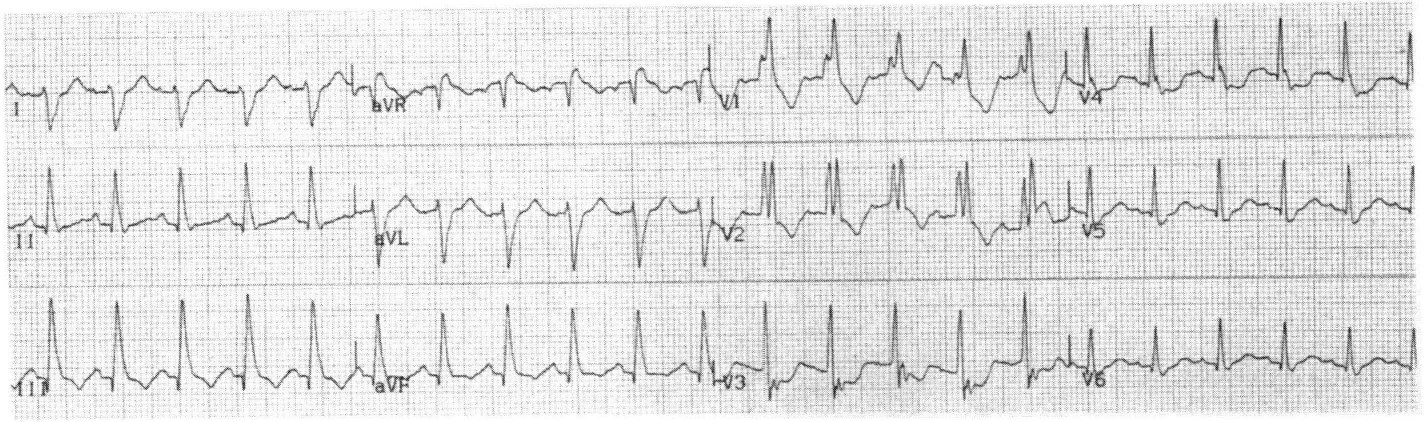

Figure 51. Left posterior fascicular block in presence of RBBB. The QRS axis is +115°.

Indeterminate or Inconsistent Frontal Plane Axis (Fig. 52)

In some cases the mean QRS vector is directed either anteriorly or posteriorly and is thus at 90° to the frontal plane. Since there is no net vector in the frontal plane, all the frontal plane leads show complexes with roughly the same amount of positive and negative deflections. The causes of an indeterminate or inconsistent frontal axis include the following:

1. Normal variant
2. S1–S2–S3 syndrome
3. Technical problems (lead misplacement)
4. Myocardial infarction
5. Right ventricular hypertrophy
6. COPD

Figure 52 shows an electrocardiogram (ECG) with an essentially indeterminate frontal axis. Figure 66 also shows an indeterminate frontal axis.

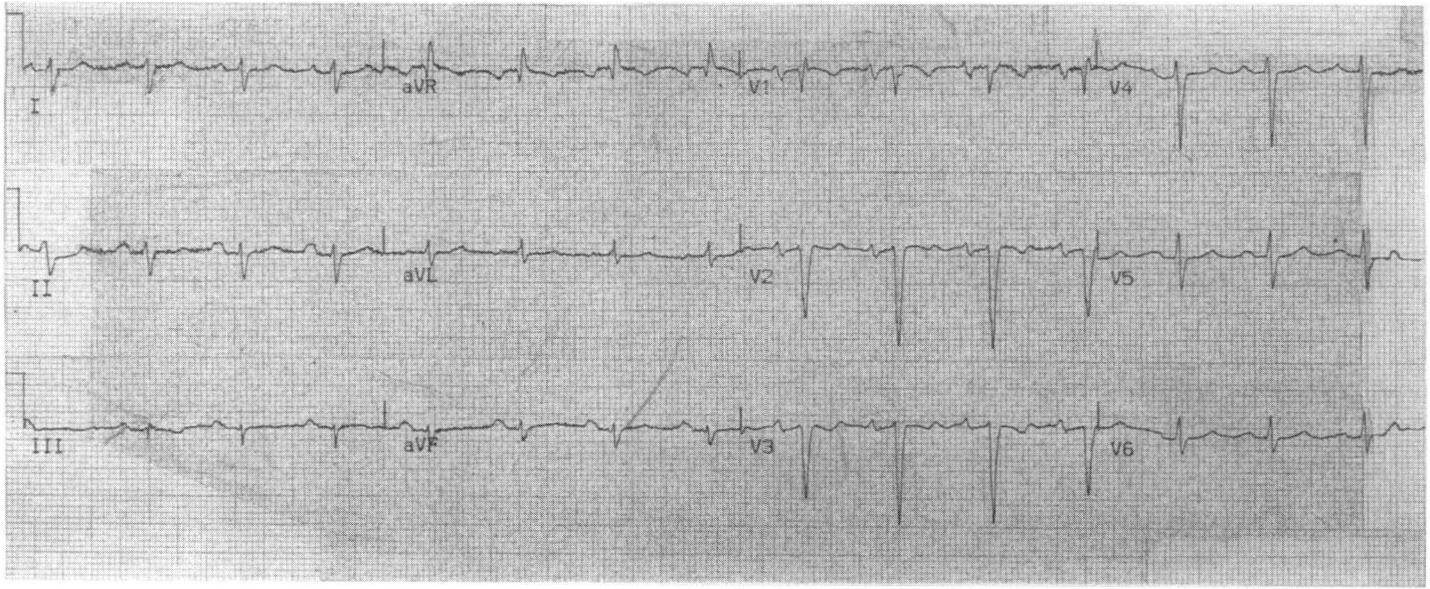

Figure 52. Electrocardiogram showing an indeterminate frontal plane axis. There is poor R-wave progression, suggesting probable anteroseptal infarction and left atrial abnormality.

Lead Placement Errors (Figs. 53–55)

Technical artifacts, most commonly lead placement errors, are a frequent cause of very abnormal ECG axis configurations. Figure 53 is a normal tracing and Figures 54 and 55 show abnormalities of axis related to lead placement. Reversals between the right and left arms are shown in Figure 54 and between the left arm and the left leg in Figure 55.

Bifascicular and Trifascicular Blocks

When two of the three conducting fascicles (right bundle branch, left anterior fascicle, and left posterior fascicle) are not conducting, bifascicular block is said to be present. Right bundle branch block (RBBB) and LAFB, or RBBB and LPFB, as shown in Figure 51, are the two disorders commonly referred to as bifascicular block.

Trifascicular block is implied when conduction is abnormal in all three fascicles, for example, in a patient with LBBB and an incomplete RBBB or a patient with bifascicular block and intermittent failure of conduction in the remaining fascicle. In practice, it is difficult to tell where the intermittent block occurs in the patient with bifascicular block and intermittent AV block, since it may occur in the AV node and not involve the third fascicle at all. Thus trifascicular block is a rather broad and ill-defined clinical entity.

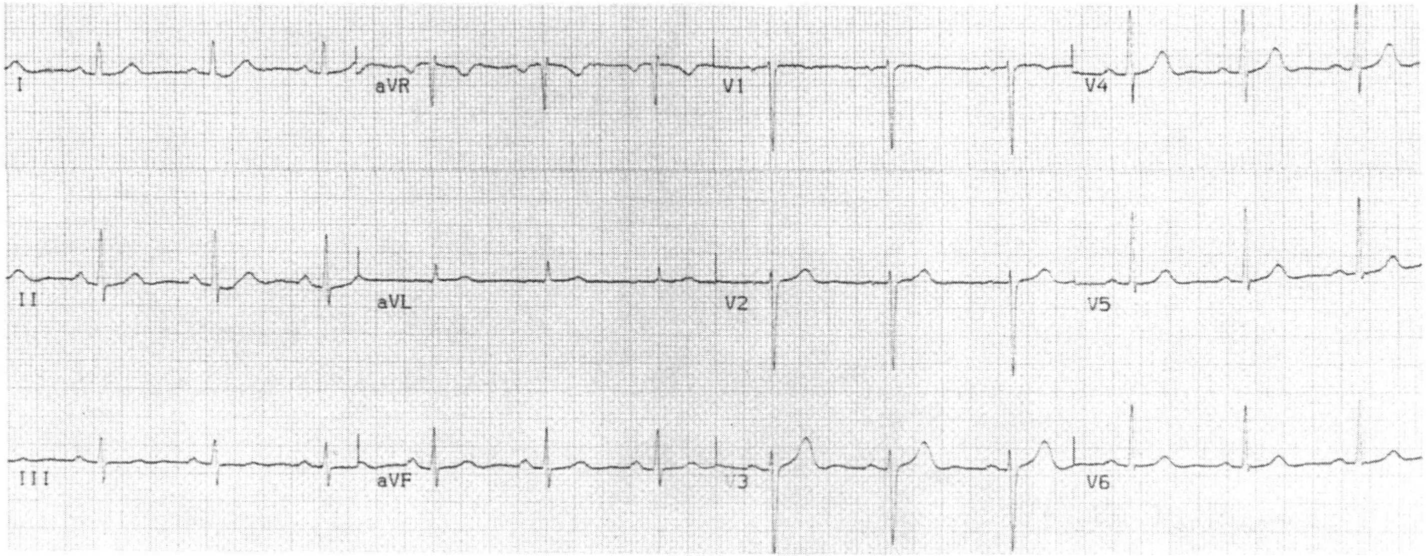

Figure 53. Normal tracing for comparison with Figures 54 and 55.

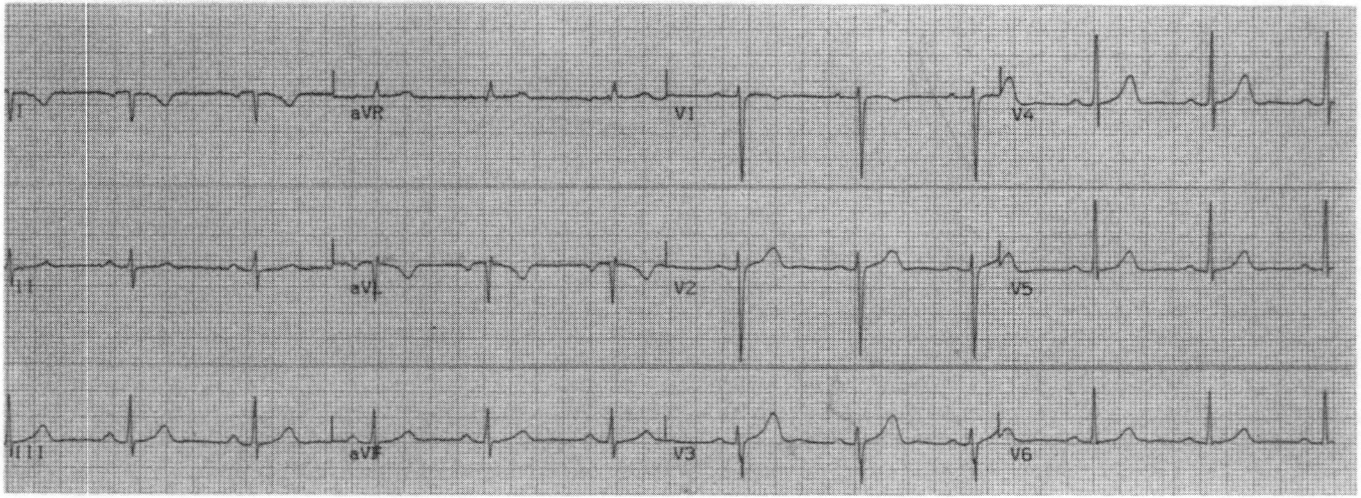

Figure 54. Reversal of right arm and left arm leads; note the simulation of far right axis deviation. The reversal of patterns in leads aVR and aVL is the most obvious tipoff to the problem. In addition, lead I is inverted and leads II and III are reversed.

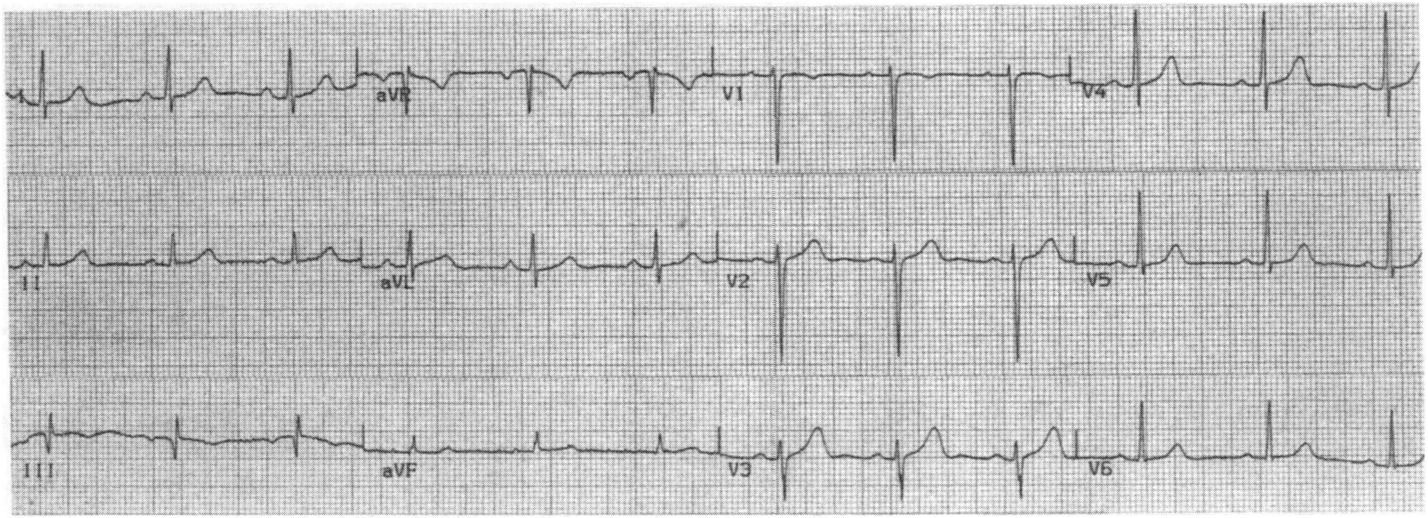

Figure 55. Reversal of left arm and left leg leads. Lead III is inverted and leads aVL and aVF as well as leads I and II are reversed.

ABNORMALITIES OF THE T-WAVE AXIS

The T-wave axis is best considered in relation to the QRS axis so that the QRS–T angle is considered. Thus, inverted T waves can be thought of as an abnormality in the T-wave axis. A difference of more than 60° between the QRS axis and the T-wave axis is suspect and one of more than 90° is abnormal, except in children. This is true for both the frontal and the horizontal plane. Abnormalities in the T-wave axis can be caused by the following conditions.

1. Normal variant
2. Abnormal depolarization pattern (e.g., LBBB, Wolff–Parkinson–White syndrome, ventricular pacing, ventricular tachycardia)
3. LVH with "strain"
4. Ischemia
5. Pericarditis
6. Many other conditions

8

Abnormalities of the P Wave

INTRODUCTION

There is a tendency to overread P-wave abnormalities, and special care should be taken to avoid unwarranted extrapolation from purely electrocardiographic (ECG) findings to physiological and anatomical inferences. For example, to state on the basis of the ECG abnormality of tall, peaked P waves in limb lead II that there is "right atrial hypertrophy" is risky indeed. It is preferable to simply state what the abnormality is and let the patient's physician decide what it means physiologically. Differences in anatomy, cardiac position, and autonomic influences all conspire to make the correlation between the P wave and the pathophysiology of the atria a poor one. Generally, the right atrium produces the first portion of the P wave, both atria produce the midportion, and the left atrium produces the terminal portion.

THE TALL P WAVE (FIG. 56)

The criteria for right atrial abnormality include a peaked P wave of 2.5 mm or more in leads II, III, and aVF. Body habitus will affect P-wave voltages in just the same manner as QRS voltages are affected. The duration should be less than 0.11 sec unless there is concomitant left atrial abnormality. Only half of the patients having this classic "P pulmonale" have actual right atrial enlargement. In the rest it represents a normal variant or left atrial abnormality. Figure 56 shows right atrial abnormality.

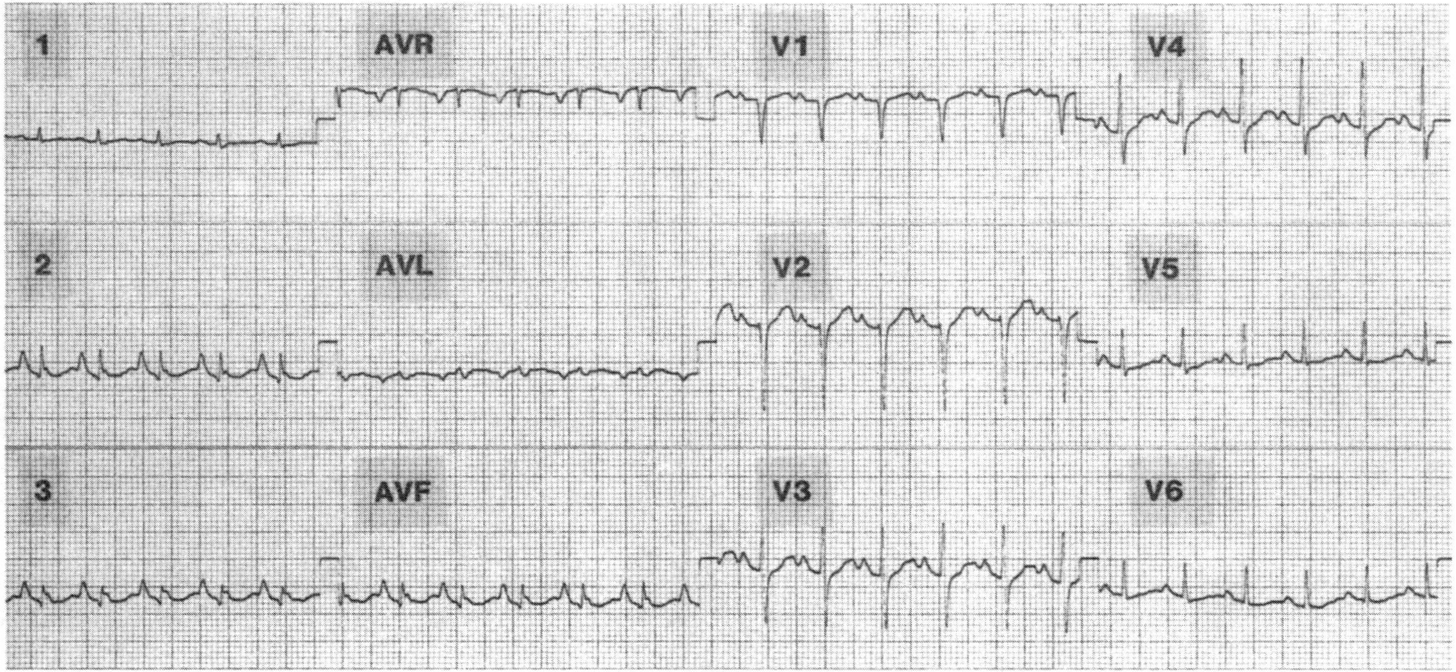

Figure 56. Right atrial abnormality. Sinus tachycardia and nonspecific ST and T changes are also present.

THE WIDE AND/OR NOTCHED P WAVE (FIG. 57)

The criteria for left atrial abnormality include a P-wave duration of over 0.10 sec (in adults), wide notching in leads I and II (>0.03 sec), and a P-wave axis leftward of +30°. It is probable that this pattern is really related to an intraatrial conduction defect rather than to anatomical "left atrial enlargement."

When atrial abnormalities occur, right and left atrial abnormalities may commonly be seen together. Figure 57 shows biatrial abnormality.

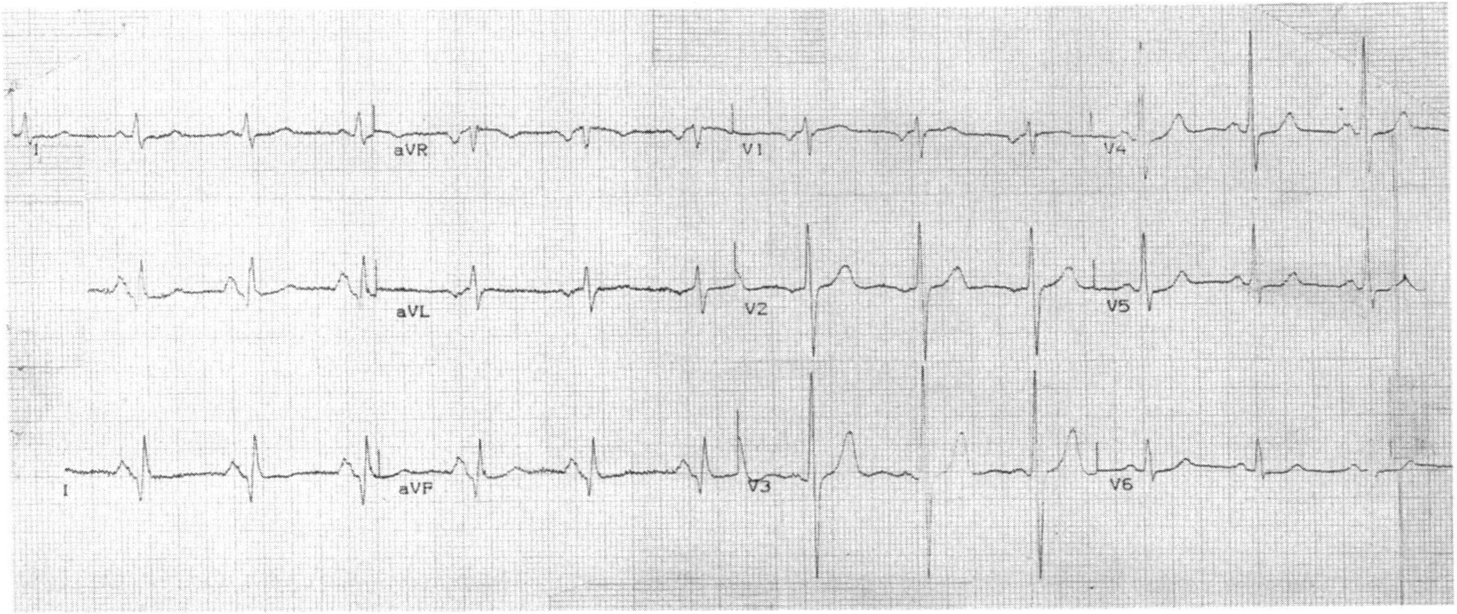

Figure 57. Biatrial enlargement. An old inferior wall myocardial infarction is also present, as shown by the Q waves in leads II, III, and AVF.

9

Abnormalities of the QRS Complex

INTRODUCTION

Abnormalities of the QRS axis and the QRS interval have been discussed in earlier chapters and will be noted in this chapter only as they relate to other problems. As a general rule, the QRS complex reflects primarily left ventricular activity and to a much lesser extent right ventricular activity, since the mass of the left ventricle is so much greater. Thus, when hypertrophy, conduction abnormalities, and infarction occur in the left ventricle, they have a much greater effect on the electrocardiogram (ECG) than when they occur in the right ventricle. Abnormalities of the right ventricle may be entirely obscured.

ABNORMALLY LOW QRS VOLTAGES

The amplitude of the QRS complex is quite dependent on a number of factors other than the myocardium. These include age, body habitus, and other factors relating to the propagation of the electrical impulse. The amplitude of the QRS voltage in at least one of the precordial leads should be greater than 10 mm and in at least one of the limb leads greater than 5 mm. The differential diagnosis of low QRS voltages includes the following conditions:

1. Normal variant
2. Obesity, anasarca
3. Chronic obstructive pulmonary disease (COPD), hyperinflation of lungs, pneumothorax
4. Effusion, pleural or pericardial
5. Diffuse myocardial disease (e.g., myocarditis, cardiomyopathy)
6. Hypothyroidism
7. Error in standardization

ABNORMALLY HIGH QRS VOLTAGES

The normal upper limits of voltage in the precordial leads, for adults over the age of 35, are an R-wave height of over 27 mm in V5 or V6; or a combined S in V1 or V2 and R in V5 or V6 of over 35 mm. In the limb leads an R wave of over 11 mm is considered abnormal. The differential diagnosis of abnormally high QRS voltages includes the following conditions.

1. Normal variant (including asthenic body build in athlete)
2. Ventricular enlargement, right or left
3. Abnormal conduction pattern (including bundle branch and fascicular blocks and accessory pathway conduction)
4. Posterior wall myocardial infarction
5. Abnormalities of body habitus, such as cachexia
6. Error in standardization

VENTRICULAR HYPERTROPHY

Introduction

The criteria for diagnosis of the ventricular hypertrophies may be unreliable, especially in borderline cases. If QRS voltage criteria are combined with the criteria of ST-segment and T-wave abnormalities, more security in the diagnosis is possible. Left ventricular hypertrophy may increase QRS duration, including the time of the intrinsicoid deflection, since the larger mass of the hypertrophied ventricle takes longer to depolarize. Age and body habitus are critical information in interpreting the ECG for evidence of hypertrophy.

Left Ventricular Hypertrophy (Figs. 58 and 59)

The diagnosis of left ventricular hypertrophy (LVH) depends more on absolute voltage values, which are, however, subject to the caveats noted earlier. A brief summary of generally accepted and more useful criteria for LVH include (in persons over the age of 30):

1. The sum of S in V1 or V2 and R in V5 or V6 is >35 mm.
2. An R-wave amplitude in any limb lead >11 mm.
3. Increased intrinsicoid deflection time to >0.05 sec in a lead with a large R wave (in the absence of any conduction defect).
4. Left ventricular strain pattern of depressed ST segments with diphasic T waves in those leads with large R-wave amplitudes.

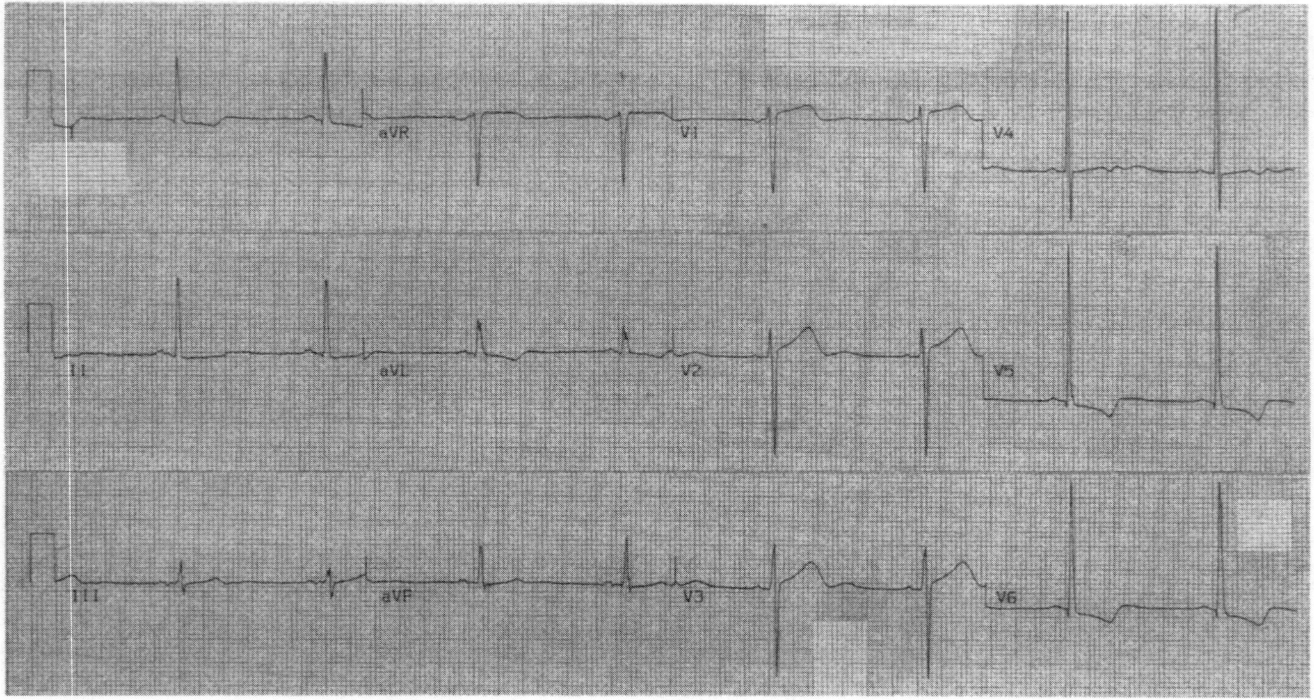

Figure 58. This tracing shows left ventricular hypertrophy with remarkable precordial voltages and left ventricular strain pattern (inverted T waves with downsloping ST segments laterally).

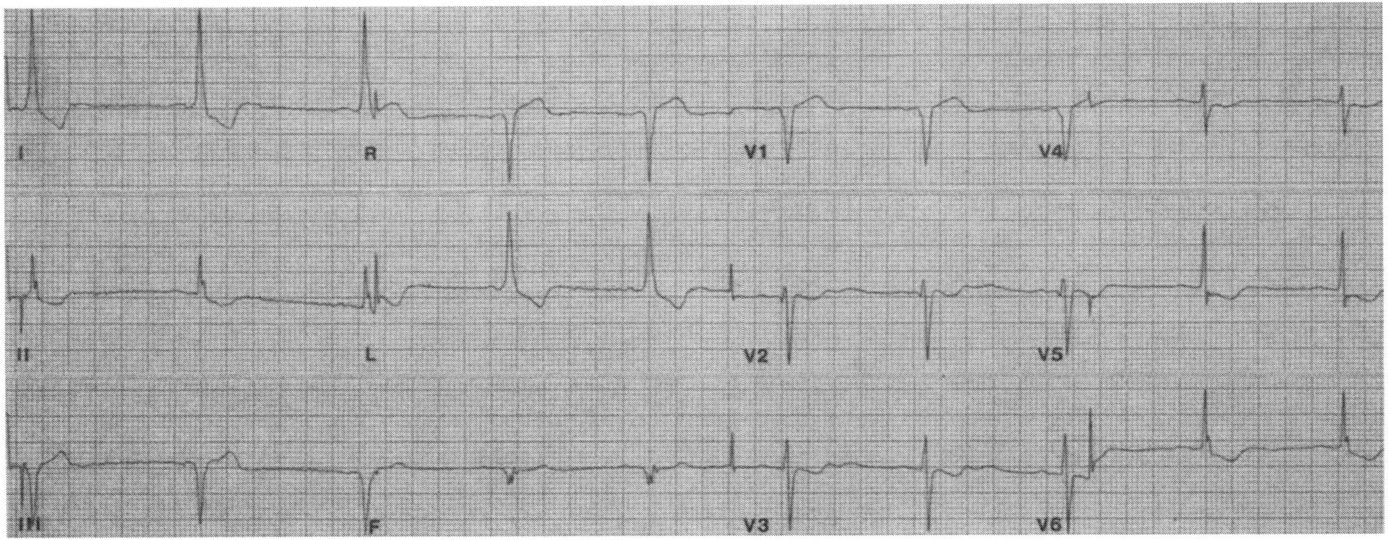

Figure 59. This tracing shows left ventricular hypertrophy without elevation of precordial voltages but with voltage increases in the limb leads and a pattern of left ventricular strain. There is also an old inferior wall infarction.

Right Ventricular Hypertrophy (Figs. 60 and 61)

Since the QRS complex is normally composed largely of left ventricular forces, an increase in the right ventricular forces will often be seen as a diminution of left ventricular forces. In addition, those leads which normally show more of the right ventricular forces will be more useful. These commonly include aVR, V1, and at times the terminal portion of the QRS in V6. It is not generally possible to distinguish between chronic right ventricular hypertrophy (RVH) and acute strain (as in cor pulmonale) without tracings taken over time. Generally, the characteristics of RVH include the following when conduction abnormalities and myocardial infarction have been ruled out. Specific voltage criteria are not helpful and the relationship between right and left ventricular forces is used to make the diagnosis. These criteria do not apply to young children.

1. R > S in V1 (or qR complex) in the absence of RBBB.
2. Prominent S in V6 (or S > R in V6).
3. Rightward axis (>110°) in the absence of a conduction defect.
4. Right-sided strain pattern, including downsloping ST segments and T-wave inversion in V1 and the inferior leads.

Figures 60 and 61 show RVH.

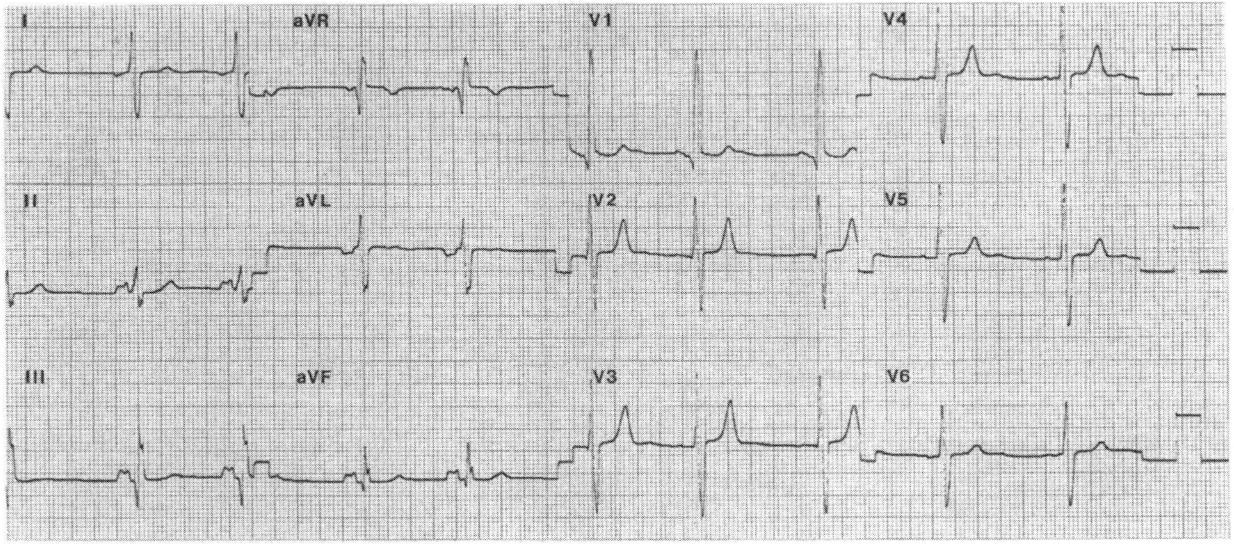

Figure 60. Tracing showing right ventricular hypertrophy. Despite the terminal R wave in aVR and the terminal S in V6 there is no true RBBB. The delay in right ventricular depolarization is due to the hypertrophied muscle mass.

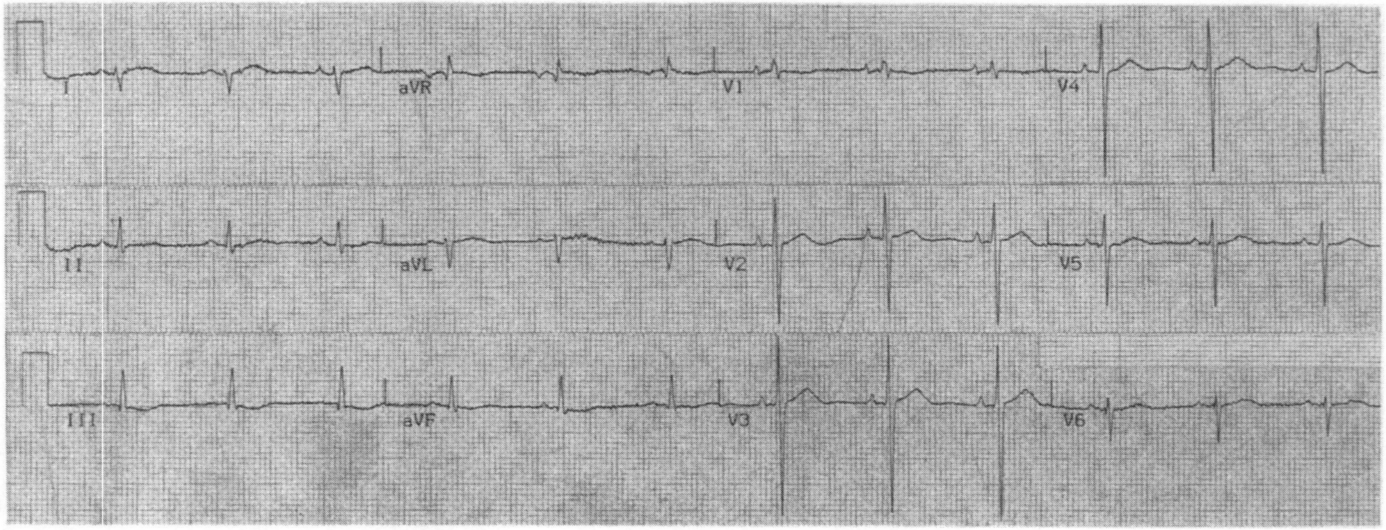

Figure 61. Tracing showing right ventricular hypertrophy. There is right-axis deviation, terminal R waves in aVR and V1, and a large S wave in V6. The axis is about +120°. The tracing is from a young patient with chronic pulmonary disease.

NORMAL AND ABNORMAL Q AND R WAVES

Introduction (Figs. 62–66)

A Q wave is an initial downward deflection of the inscription of the QRS complex. Q waves occur normally in some ECG leads, and it is important to distinguish normal from abnormal Q waves, since abnormal Q waves are the hallmark of myocardial infarction and both overdiagnosis and underdiagnosis can cause the patient harm. Normal Q waves resulting from septal activity are commonly seen in the lateral precordial leads and in I and aVL. A Q wave is also common in aVR, since that lead "looks into" the cavity of the left ventricle. Similarly, Q waves may occur normally in V1 and even V2 if these leads are looking mainly at the inside of the left ventricle. A Q wave can be seen normally in lead 3. In fact, the complete absence of septal Qs in I, aVL, V5, and V6 raises the question of septal fibrosis or infarction. Relatively prominent Q waves can also result from the conduction disturbances found in the fascicular blocks (see discussions of left anterior and left posterior fascicular block, Chapter 7).

Abnormal Q waves occur as a result of myocardial infarction or septal hypertrophy, the former being much more common. When they occur as the result of infarction, they are broad (0.04 sec or more) and relatively deeper than "normal" Q waves—more than 25% of the height of the accompanying R wave. Pathological Qs should be present in more than one related lead (e.g., II as well as III, I as well as aVL) to be considered abnormal and indicative of myocardial infarction. At times the Q may be present only as its "equivalent," that is, a larger-than-expected R wave in V1 representing the equivalent of the Q of a posterior myocardial infarction, or as a reduced R wave in the precordial leads. As a general rule, isolated Qs have less meaning than widespread ones. Q waves occurring in older persons and persons with other evidence of cardiac pathology are also more suspect.

Abnormal Q waves begin to be seen within minutes to hours after myocardial infarction. The location of the ECG changes seen following myocardial infarction follows logically from a knowledge of the areas that each lead looks at. As noted earlier, the loss of electrical forces due to infarction may be seen as a Q wave, as a loss of normal R wave, or as the presence of a larger-than-normal R wave when the infarction is seen by a lead looking from the opposite side of the infarcted area. The following patterns can commonly be seen.

1. Q waves in the inferior leads (II, III, and aVF) suggest inferior wall infarction.
2. Q waves in the superior or high lateral leads (I, aVL) suggest superior or high lateral infarction.
3. Q waves, poor R-wave progression, or decreasing R wave in the mid-precordium (V2, V3, V4) suggests anterior wall infarction. There may be an associated absence of septal Qs in the lateral precordial leads (V5, V6) if the septum was involved.
4. Q waves and abnormally decreased R waves in the lateral precordial leads (V5, V6) and possibly the superior leads (I, aVL) suggest lateral wall or apical infarction.
5. A large R wave (R greater than S) with a duration of greater than 0.04 sec in V1 suggests true posterior wall infarction.

Figures 43 and 44 show inferior Q waves which are small and normal—no infarction is suggested. By comparison, Figure 62 has inferior wall Q waves that are larger and abnormal, and are diagnostic of inferior wall myocardial infarction. Other common patterns of myocardial infarction are shown in Figure 63 (anterior), Figure 64 (posterior), Figure 65 (lateral), and Figure 66 (anterosuperior).

The absence of Q waves does not go far toward disproving infarction since as many as 15–30% of persons with documented transmural myocardial infarctions may lose their Q waves over time. Nontransmural infarctions generally have no Q wave present at all. The presence of left anterior fascicular block can on occasion mask the Qs of inferior infarction.

Right ventricular infarctions also occur, but are hard to detect electrocardiographically owing to the small contribution of the right ventricular forces to the ECG.

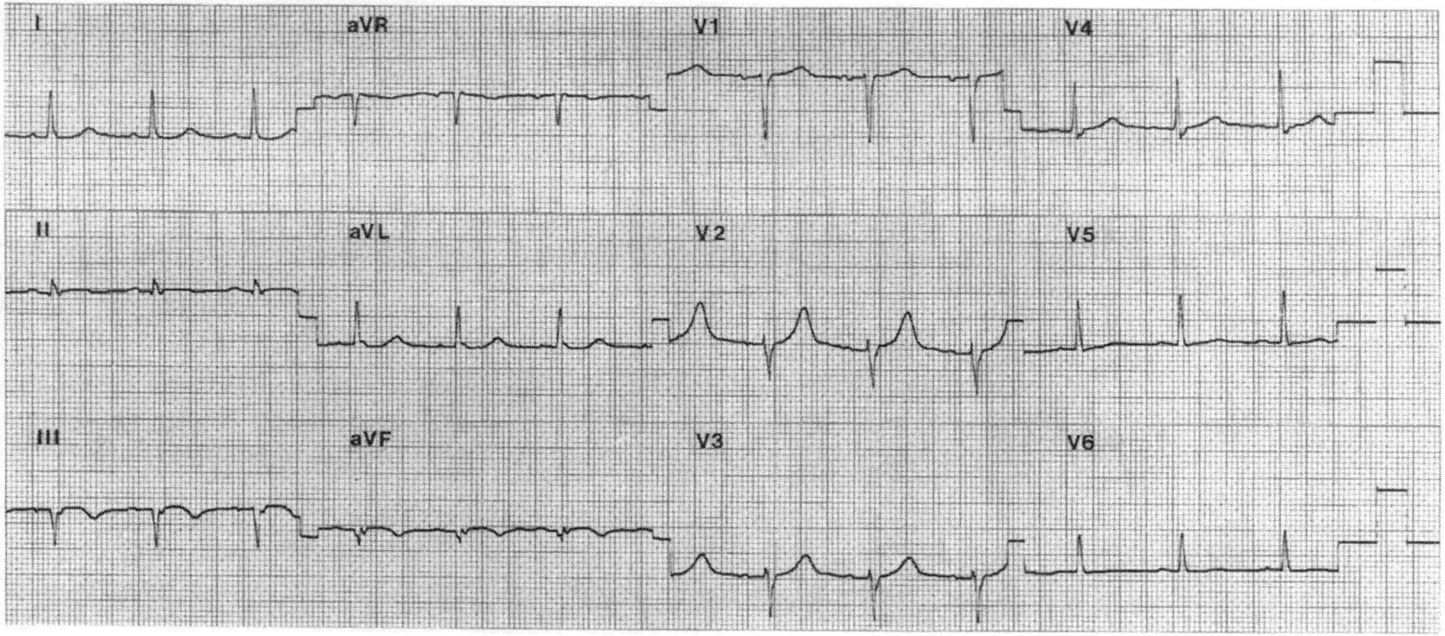

Figure 62. The inferior wall Q waves with persistent T-wave inversion are evidence of inferior myocardial infarction.

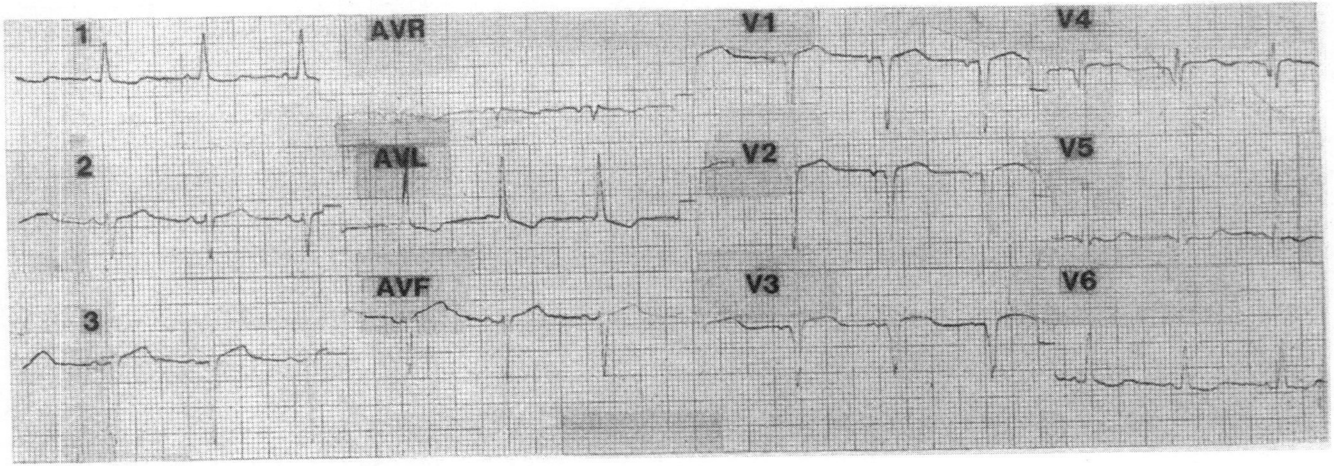

Figure 63. Anterior wall myocardial infarction is indicated by QS complexes in V1 through V3 and a large Q in V4. Anterior and inferior ST-segment depression is also present, and the axis is −50°, suggesting LAFB.

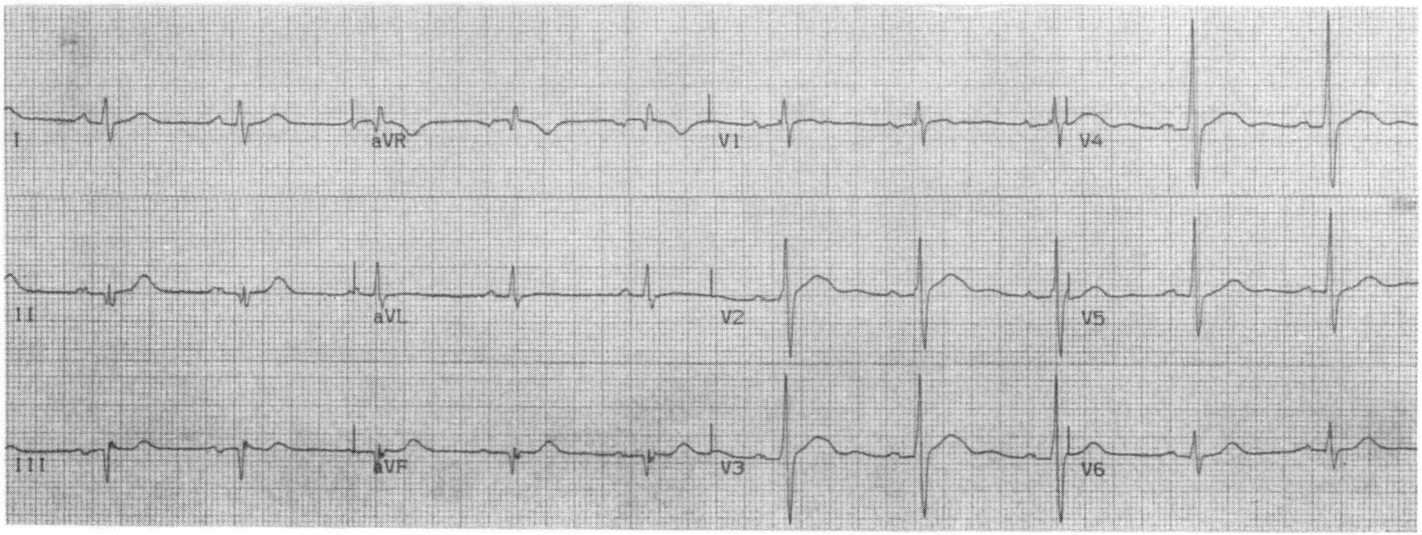

Figure 64. True posterior myocardial infarction is suggested by large R waves in V1 and V2 (really Q waves "seen" from the opposite side of the heart). Inferior Q waves are also present, as is commonly seen with true posterior infarctions.

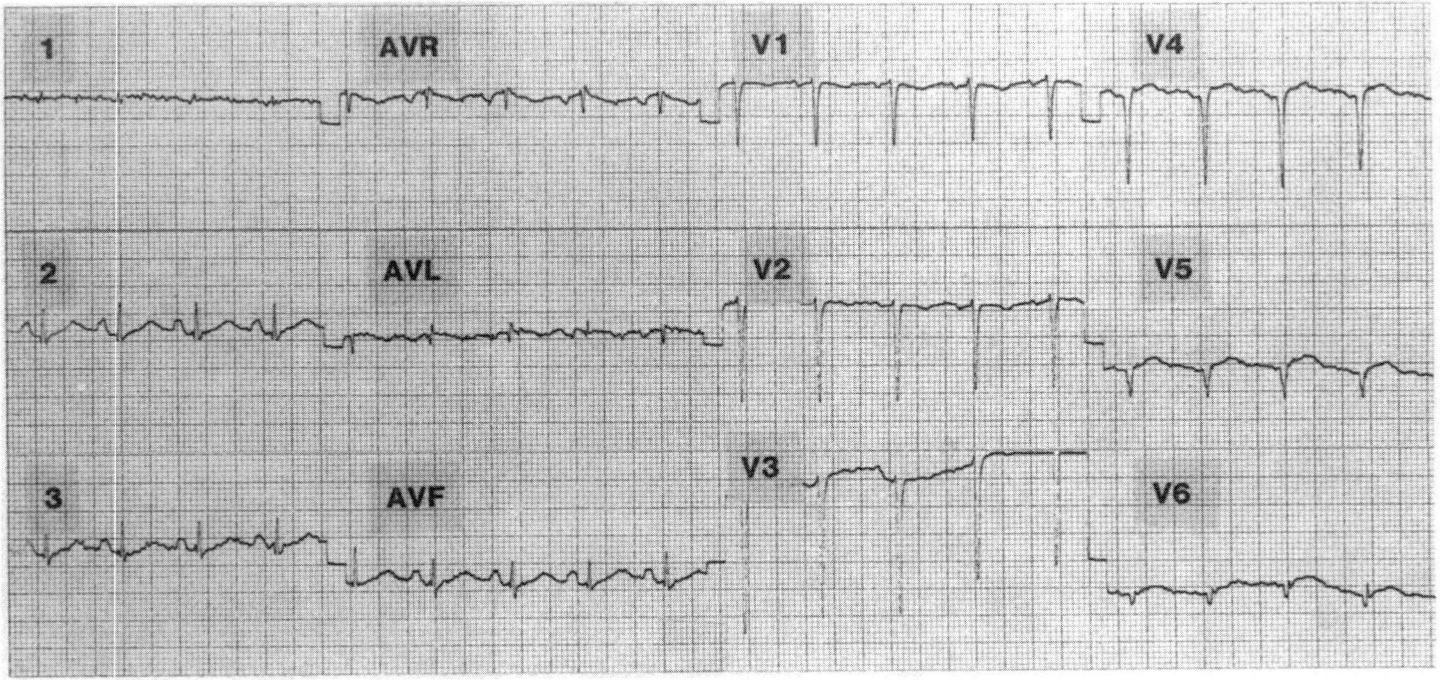

Figure 65. Lateral wall myocardial infarction. QS complexes or large Q waves are seen in V4 through V6.

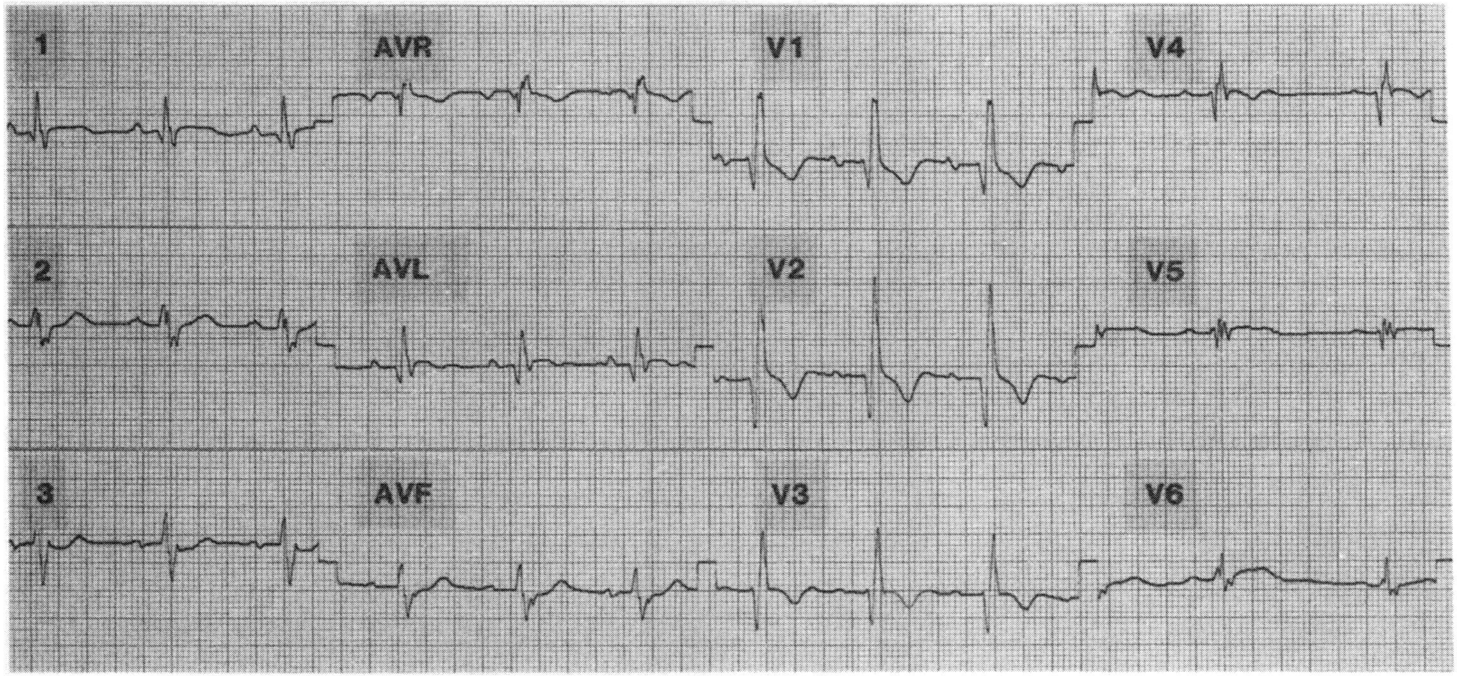

Figure 66. Anterosuperior infarction is present based on the Q waves in I, aVL, and V1–V4. Right bundle branch block is also present, as is first-degree AV block. The frontal plane axis is indeterminate.

Causes of Pseudoinfarction Patterns

Unfortunately, the presence of Q waves is not always specific for myocardial infarction, since a number of other conditions can give rise to abnormal Q waves, abnormal R waves, or poor R-wave progression. These include the patterns shown in Table 3.

Accessory Pathway Syndromes (Fig. 67)

A wide variety of conduction disturbances, pseudoinfarction patterns, and rhythm disturbances are related to the accessory pathway syndromes, most commonly seen as the Wolff–Parkinson–White (WPW) syndromes. In this syndrome there is a short

Table 3. Causes of Abnormal Q Waves, R Waves, and Poor R-Wave Progression

1. Q waves in the inferior leads suggesting inferior infarction
   - A. Normal variant (if small)
   - B. LBBB
   - C. WPW
   - D. COPD
   - E. RVH
   - F. Technical error (lead misplacement)
2. Q waves, QS complexes in right precordium, poor R-wave progression suggesting anterior or anteroseptal infarction
   - A. Normal variant
   - B. Left anterior fascicular block
   - C. LBBB or ILBBB
   - D. WPW
   - E. RVH
   - F. LVH
   - G. COPD, cor pulmonale
   - H. Diffuse myocardial disease (e.g., amyloidosis)
   - I. Dextrocardia, pectus excavatum, pneumothorax
   - J. Technical error (smeared electrode paste)
3. Q waves in superior (I, aVL) and/or lateral leads suggesting superior or lateral wall infarction
   - A. Normal (if small and "septal")
   - B. Technical (limb-lead reversal causes Q in I)
   - C. Septal hypertrophy (e.g., IHSS, LVH)
4. Tall and/or broad R wave in V1 suggesting true posterior infarction
   - A. Normal variant
   - B. RBBB, IRBBB
   - C. WPW
   - D. RVH
   - E. IHSS and other cardiomyopathies

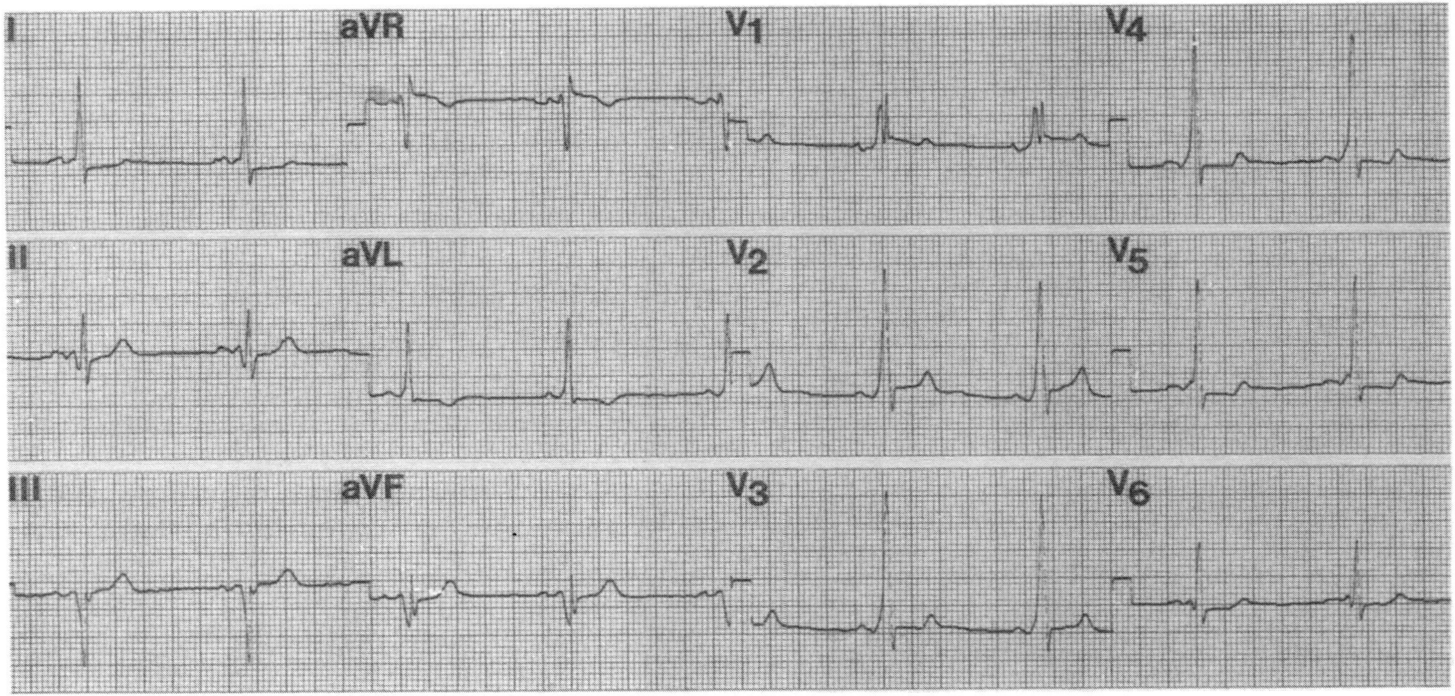

Figure 67. Wolff–Parkinson–White syndrome with conduction pattern simulating inferior wall myocardial infarction. Compare Figure 7.

P–R interval (less than 0.12 sec) and slurring of the upstroke of the QRS complex by a delta wave, caused by preexcitation of the ventricles over the accessory pathway prior to conduction over the normal conducting system. Figure 67 shows an ECG during sinus rhythm of a patient with the WPW syndrome. Many different configurations of the ECG are possible in the WPW syndrome, depending on the precise anatomical location of the accessory pathway.

Poor R-Wave Progression

This is a relatively common ECG finding which may occur in 10% of a hospitalized population. The heart is normal in nearly 40% of the cases, with a similar number due to anterior myocardial infarction and the remainder split almost equally between RVH and LVH.[4] In persons with COPD the poor R-wave progression may be due to a combination of an abnormal chest configuration and RVH.

Other Variations of the QRS Complex

RSR′ patterns may be seen in the anterior precordium in normal individuals, sometimes with small terminal R waves in aVR as a manifestation of late activation of the posterior septum. In addition, abnormalities of the intervals, axis, or voltages may be seen, especially in well-conditioned younger patients.

10

Abnormalities of the ST Segment

INTRODUCTION

The ST segment is the period between the cessation of the QRS complex which is marked by the J point and the onset of the T wave. In interpretation of the ST segment, the shape (concave or convex upward) and the slope are sometimes as important as the absolute degree of ST-segment elevation or depression. Associated T-wave changes are also important. The large number of factors affecting the ST segment often makes interpretation difficult. In addition, the relative lack of sensitivity of the ST segment for ischemia and infarction means that clinical decisions regarding the care of a patient with suspected ischemia and/or infarction must be made on clinical grounds if the electrocardiogram is normal. Normal ST segments do not rule out ischemia, infarction, or other conditions.

ELEVATED ST SEGMENTS (Figs. 68–70)

To be significant the elevation should be 1 mm or greater. The ST-segment changes associated with myocardial injury tend to be convex upward or flattened. The ST-segment elevation that is occasionally seen in normal individuals (normal early repolarization pattern) is typically concave upward, the T wave is tall and normal, and the ST axis is typically in the same direction as the T-wave axis. Some of the causes of ST segment elevation are the following.

1. Normal early repolarization pattern
2. Myocardial injury during the course of acute myocardial infarction
3. Myocardial injury during acute coronary artery spasm (variant or Prinzmetal's angina)
4. Ventricular aneurysm following myocardial infarction (this may result in ST-segment elevation which persists for years)
5. Pericarditis and myocarditis
6. Conduction abnormalities
7. Multiple central nervous system, endocrine, and other causes (rarely)

Figures 68 and 69 show tall, peaked T waves, and ST-segment elevation occurring early during the course of an anteroseptal myocardial infarction, compared with a tracing taken a few hours later. Figure 70 shows typical ST-segment elevation in an acute inferior wall infarction.

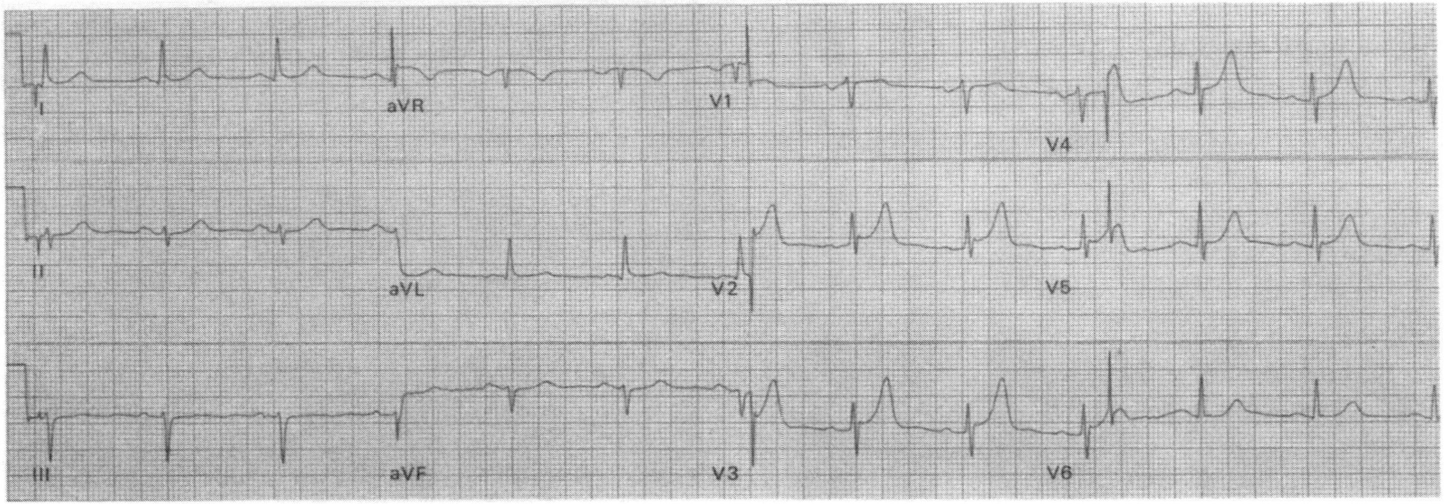

Figure 68. Tall, peaked, "hyperacute" T waves with early anteroseptal infarction. This patient progressed to a typical myocardial infarction over the next several hours. On this tracing, Q waves have not yet developed. Left-axis deviation with probable LAFB is also present.

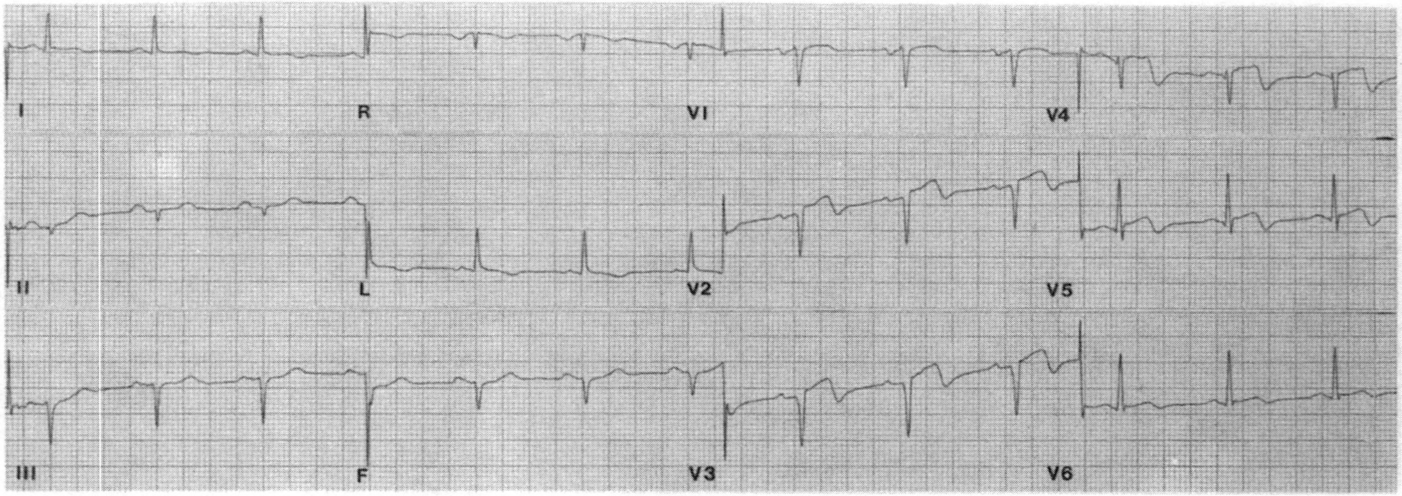

Figure 69. The same patient as in Figure 68. This electrocardiogram was taken a few hours later. The T waves are now inverted, and the ST-segment elevation is more pronounced. Q waves have appeared, confirming the presence of acute myocardial infarction.

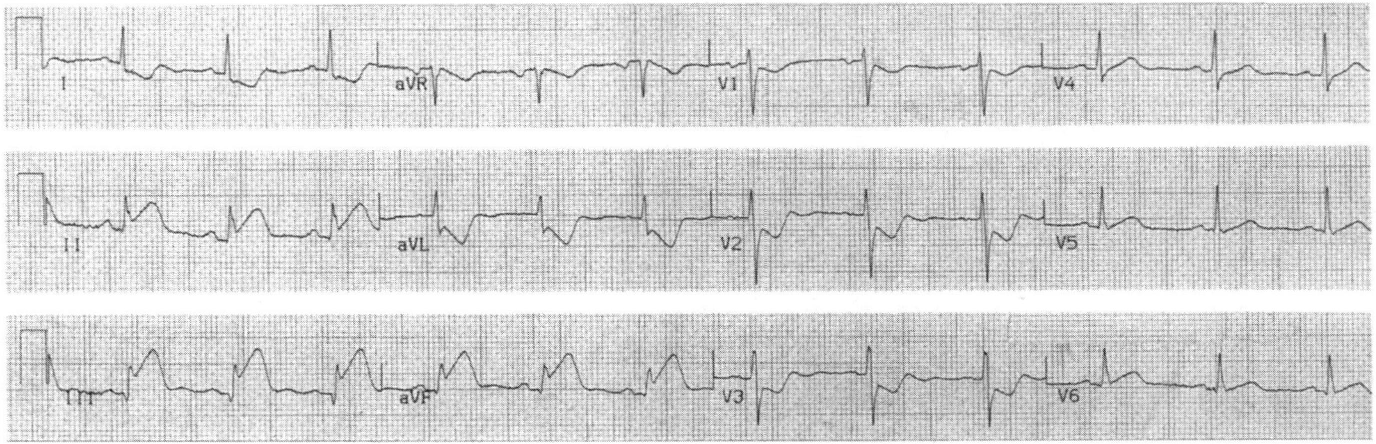

Figure 70. Typical ST–T wave changes over the inferior wall in a patient with an acute inferior wall infarction. There is inferior ST segment elevation, Q waves are just starting to develop, and there are reciprocal changes in the anterior and lateral leads.

DEPRESSED ST SEGMENTS

To be significant the depression should usually be 1 mm or greater. "Normal" ST-segment depression is less common than "normal" ST-segment elevation, but nonetheless can occur. One apparent cause of ST-segment depression is the Tp wave (also called the Ta wave), which is the equivalent of the T wave resulting from atrial repolarization. This is most prominent during exercise or in persons with large P waves. Note that the depression of the ST segment forms a nearly perfect semicircle with the PQ segment. The causes of ST-segment depression include the following.

1. Nonspecific changes
2. Hyperventilation
3. Conduction abnormalities
4. Ventricular strain (right or left)
5. Tachycardia
6. Tp (Ta) Wave
7. Ischemia and subendocardial infarction
8. Changes reciprocal to ST-segment elevation in an opposite lead
9. Digitalis
10. Hypokalemia
11. Cerebral disease (especially intracerebral hemorrhage)

Figure 71 shows a diagram of ST-segment changes due to strain, ischemia, digitalis, Tp wave, and normal variants.

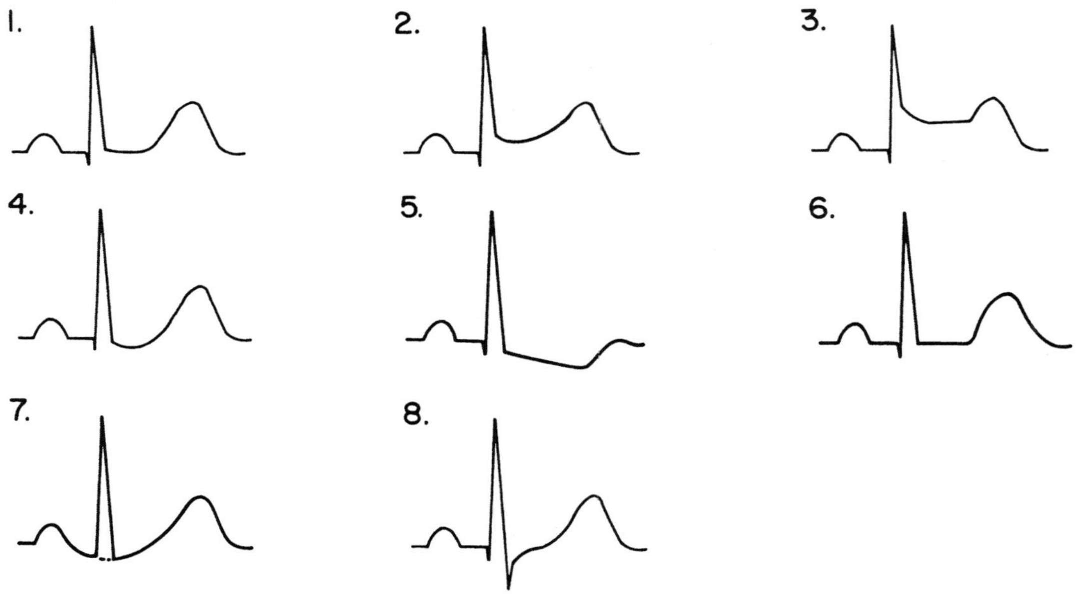

Figure 71. Various ST-segment configurations. (1) Normal. The ST segment is slightly rounded. (2) Common normal variant, especially seen in anterior precordial leads. Tends to be concave upward. (3) ST-segment elevation due to injury such as ischemic injury or pericarditis. It tends to be flat to concave downward and to occur in a more widespread fashion. (4) ST-segment sagging as occurs with digitalis. Note that the contour is somewhat rounded—that is, it sags! (5) ST-segment depression due to strain and/or ischemia. The ST segment is flatter, less rounded, and downsloping with a sharper angle at the transition to the T wave. (6) ST segment showing isoelectric flattening suggestive of ischemia. Normally the ST segment is slightly rounded and the level flattening suggests ischemia. (7) ST-segment depression due to Ta wave (the T wave resulting from atrial repolarization). Note that the Ta wave describes nearly a circular arc from the P wave to the T wave. (8) ST-segment depression due to normal J-point depression, the J point being the transition between the termination of the QRS complex and the ST segment. The ST segment is clearly upsloping.

11

Abnormalities of the T Wave and the U Wave

INTRODUCTION

The T wave is even more susceptible to a variety of influences than the ST segment and thus is less reliable as a marker of pathological or physiological derangement since the majority of T-wave abnormalities are nonspecific. The T-wave axis in the frontal plane may differ from the QRS axis by as much as 50° before abnormality is present. T waves may be normal even in the presence of ischemia or infarction. Alterations in the T wave are common in children with diphasic or notched T waves in the anterior precordium being the most common pattern (see Figure 72). T-wave abnormalities may be of two types. There may be primary changes in repolarization due to ischemia or metabolic problems or changes in the sequence of depolarization, as is the case with conduction abnormalities. The characteristics of normal T waves are the following:

1. Inverted in aVR and frequently V1
2. Upright in I, II, and the lateral precordial leads
3. Variable in leads III, aVL, and aVF (if QRS voltage is low) and in leads V1 and V2 and sometimes V3
4. Axis within 50° of QRS axis
5. Less than 5 mm in limb leads and 10 mm in precordial leads
6. Rounded and slightly asymmetrical contour

THE T WAVE IN MYOCARDIAL INFARCTION

The first T-wave changes in acute myocardial infarction usually include, along with the ST-segment elevation, some increase in T-wave amplitude ("hyperacute T waves") or early T-wave inversion. Typically, during the course of evolution of myocardial infarction, the ST segments remain elevated for a matter of hours to days, and during this period, the T waves become inverted. This T-wave inversion typically persists for far longer than the ST-segment elevation, and the T waves may remain inverted for months or years after infarction. However, variations on this scenario are common and may consist of early

ST-segment depression (less common than elevation) and inconsistent T-wave changes which may persist for life. Figures 66 and 68–70 show T-wave changes in infarction.

TALL T WAVES

The differential diagnosis of the tall T wave, which to be considered as abnormal should be both symmetrical and peaked, includes the following conditions. Figure 68 shows tall T waves due to early infarction.

1. Normal variant or nonspecific changes
2. Acute myocardial infarction or ischemia
3. Hyperkalemia
4. Left ventricular hypertrophy (LVH)
5. Changes reciprocal to deep T-wave inversion in an opposite lead (e.g., on the right precordium for true posterior wall infarction)

DIPHASIC OR INVERTED T WAVES (FIG. 72)

The T-wave changes seen in acute myocardial ischemia can occur immediately or be delayed for hours to days. T-wave changes are not reliable indicators of infarction, although a pattern of changing T waves may be. When T-wave changes are associated with infarction, they tend to take the form of symmetrical T-wave inversion. The causes of diphasic or inverted T waves are as follows:

1. Normal, juvenile T pattern, nonspecific changes
2. Myocardial ischemia and/or infarction
3. Abnormal conduction patterns
4. Ventricular hypertrophy ("strain"), right or left
5. Myocarditis, pericarditis
6. Electrolyte disorders
7. Drugs
8. Cerebral disease (especially acute intracerebral hemorrhage, which can cause deep, symmetrical T-wave inversions and Q–T interval prolongation)

Figure 72 shows the symmetrical T-wave inversion of ischemia across the anterior precordium. The tracing also shows LVH.

ABNORMALITIES OF THE U WAVE

The normal U wave is small and in the same direction as the preceding T wave. It is altered by a number of factors and is more prominent with bradycardic rhythms, hypokalemia, and LVH. The enlarged U wave in patients with hypokalemia can give the impression of a prolonged Q–T interval.

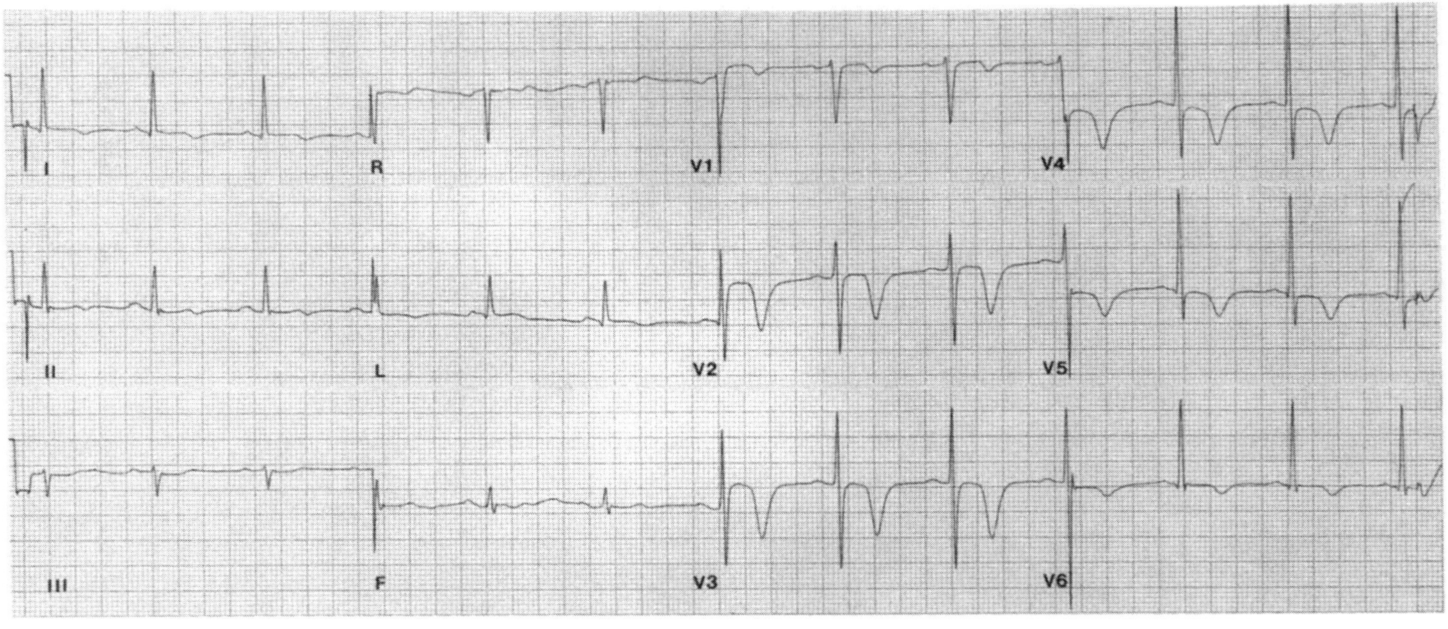

Figure 72. Symmetrical T-wave inversion strongly suggestive of acute ischemia in the anterior precordial leads. This could also be seen with acute intracranial hemorrhage. The tracing also shows left ventricular hypertrophy.

12

The Electrocardiogram in Childhood

INTRODUCTION

The differences in electrocardiograms (ECGs) between infants and adults relate to the relative sizes of the right and left ventricles, the normal heart rate, and conduction differences related to the physical size of the heart. In addition, high voltages may be seen because of the thin chest wall. Patterns of repolarization that would be abnormal in an adult are quite common in children and may persist into the teens and occasionally beyond.

QRS AXIS

At birth the average QRS axis is greater than $+130°$, with a prominent R wave in the right precordial leads. Within a few days to a month the QRS axis moves into a range (less than $+110°$) that would be considered normal, though still rightward, for adults. By age 6 years a prominent initial R wave in V1 remains common, although the QRS pattern in the ECG should otherwise be quite similar to that of the adult. An R′ may be seen in the right precordial leads (along with a normal-length QRS) as a normal pattern, probably resulting from late depolarization of the posterior septum. The diagnosis of ventricular hypertrophy in children requires the use of detailed age-specific tables of criteria, which can be found in more detailed texts.

ST SEGMENTS

ST-segment elevation in the precordial leads, usually with upward coving of the ST segment, is common. The elevation may be from 2 to 4 mm. This pattern may persist into adult life but becomes less common.

T WAVES (FIG. 73)

There are several variations of the T waves which relate in part to large differences in the T wave and the QRS axis. Thus, T-wave inversion is common; in addition, diphasic T waves are also common, as are patterns of notching of the T's, which may even simulate extra P waves.

Figure 73 shows the peculiar T waves occasionally found in children.

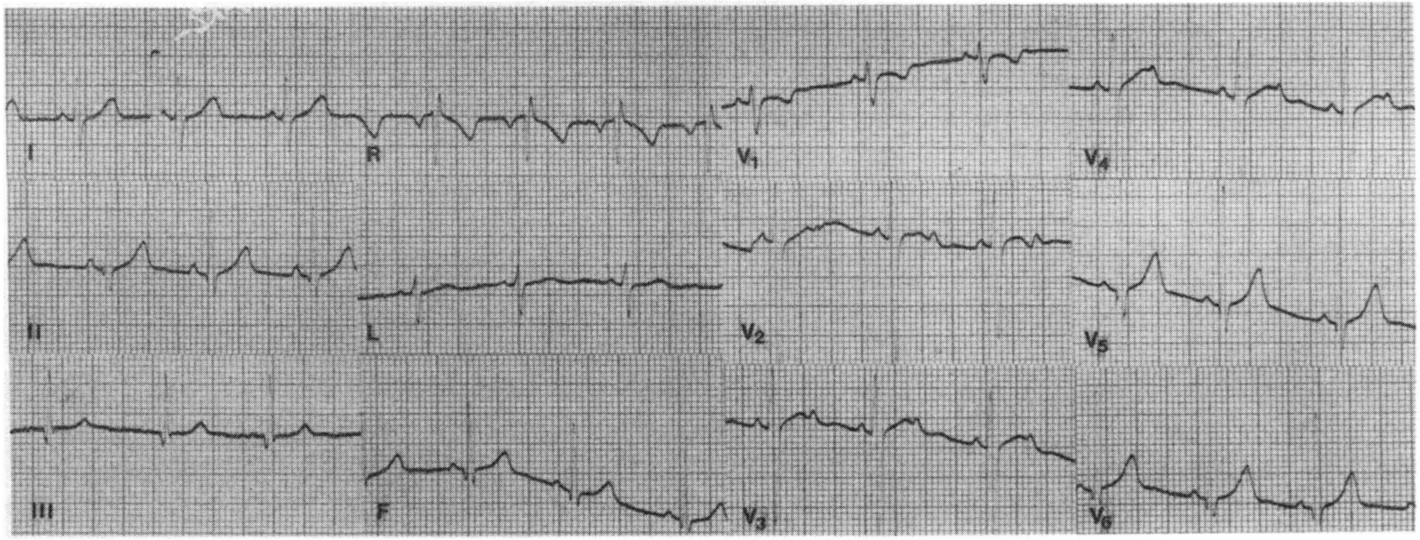

Figure 73. Normal T waves in an 8-year-old child. This tracing may be mistaken for 2:1 atrioventricular block based on the pattern in the precordial leads. This is not the case, as suggested by the fact that the ventricular rate does not change significantly despite the apparent block and the apparent "P" waves in the precordial leads do not march out in a regular fashion.

References

1. Friedman, HH: *Diagnostic Electrocardiography and Vectorcardiography,* ed. 3. New York, McGraw-Hill, 1985.
2. Wharton JM, Goldschlager N: *Guide to Interpreting 12-Lead ECG's.* Oradell, NJ, Medical Economics Books, 1984.
3. Grauer K, Curry RW: *Clinical Electrocardiography—A Primary Care Approach.* Oradell, NJ, Medical Economics Books, 1987.
4. Goldman MJ: *Principles of Clinical Electrocardiography,* ed. 11. Los Altos, CA, Lange Medical Publications, 1986.
5. Marriott HJ: *Practical Electrocardiography,* ed. 8. Baltimore, Williams & Wilkins, 1988.
6. Sox HC, Margulies I, Sox CH: Psychologically mediated effects of diagnostic tests. *Ann Intern Med* 1981;95:680–685.
7. Fisch C: Abnormal ECG in clinically normal individuals. *JAMA* 1983;150:1321–1323.
8. Kapoor WN, Karpf M, Wieand S, Peterson JR, Levey GS. A prospective evaluation and follow-up of patients with syncope. *N Engl J Med* 1983;309:197–204.
9. Kapoor WN, Karpf M, Levey GS. Issues in evaluating patients with syncope. *Ann Intern Med* 1984;100:755–757.
10. Josephson ME, Seides SF. *Clinical Cardiac Electrophysiology:*

Techniques and Interpretations. Philadelphia, Lea & Febiger, 1979.

11. Rahilly GT, Prystowski EN, Zipes DP, Naccarelli GV, Jackman WM, Heger JJ. Clinical and electrophysiologic findings in patients with repetitive monomorphic ventricular tachycardia and otherwise normal electrocardiogram. *Am J Cardiol* 1982;50:459–468.
12. Wellens HJJ, Barr FWHM, Lie KI. The value of the electrocardiogram in the differential diagnosis of a tachycardia with a widened QRS complex. *Am J Med* 1978;64:27–33.
13. Moss AJ. Prolonged QT-interval syndromes. *JAMA* 1986;256:2985–2987.
14. Zema MJ, Kligfield P. ECG poor R-wave progression, review and synthesis. *Arch Intern Med* 1982;142:1145–1148.

Index

Italicized page numbers indicate figures.

About the Authors

John W. Beasley, M.D., is board-certified by the American Board of Family Practice. He is Associate Professor of Family Medicine and Practice at the University of Wisconsin Medical School and Associate Chairman of the Department of Family Medicine and Practice.

E. Wayne Grogan, Jr., M.D., is board-certified by the American Board of Internal Medicine in Internal Medicine and Cardiovascular Disease. He is Assistant Professor of Medicine at the University of Wisconsin Medical School and Director of Cardiac Electrophysiology at the University of Wisconsin Hospital and Clinics.